Moderr
Electrology:

Excess Hair, Its Causes and Treatments - Including Laser

By Fino Gior

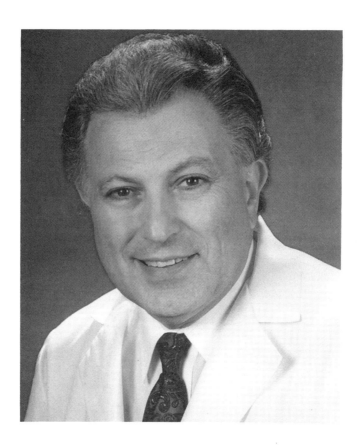

Hair Publishing, Inc.
Medical Center   15 Bond Street   Suite 111
Great Neck, New York 11021

Editorial Director:	Mary Healy
Associate Editor:	May Jane Tenerelli
Consultant:	Bobbi Ray Madry
Art Director:	John Patric Fornieri
Illustrator:	Shiz Horil
Editorial Assistant:	Ken Morris
Production Assistant:	Kisa Molinari
Phototypesetter:	Paul Gafton
Graphic Artist:	Pat Genova, Pat Miret, Mark Stein

Hair Publishing—Fourth Edition 2005— First 1987, Copyright
Printed in the United States of America

Foreword

The publication of *Modern Electrology* stands as a milestone in the field of electrology.

Recent years have seen a growing demand for professional training, validated by licensure or, at the very least, a certification examination. *Modern Electrology* provides the first comprehensive text covering all aspects of this emerging field.

The purpose of this book is to educate men and women in the profession of electrology, preparing them for licensure or certification, serving also as a reference guide for the graduate electrologist and associated professionals.

Modern Electrology fully explains and illustrates the knowledge and skills the professional electrologist must possess to be a success.

- The textbook was designed to give the student a thorough understanding of the theory and practice of all the pertinent subjects dealing with the process of permanent hair removal.
- The complete course of study allows for flexibility so that instructors and students can adapt the material to the techniques they find most practical and effective.
- Margin headings identify key subject matter and enhance concentrated study.
- Each chapter is a complete unit of study that can be shortened or lenghtened to meet the needs of personalized lesson plans.
- Safety symbols flag key items for safety and protection of the public.
- An extensive glossary of terms, illustrations, charts, and photos further aids the instructor and the student. Learning objectives begin each chapter, and questions are provided to evaluate if those objectives are met.
- The contents are arranged in a logical sequence for instruction. Schools or instructors may alter the sequence to fit their curriculum.
- Graduating students will be better prepared for their state board examinations and certification programs where applicable.

Important Message From The Author

I have been a full time practicing electrologist for 42 years. This book contains the knowledge and experience of those years, which I wish to share with the new student, the public as well as the practicing electrologists.

The profession of electrology is dedicated in making people happy. I have seen many, many times the distress that so many of my patients, male and female, suffer from the disfigurement of excess hair on their face or body. To be able to relieve this distress for an individual is most satisfying to the patient as well as to the practitioner and it is forever. This is true success not just making money.

A career in electrology requires a particular talent, sincere and honest concern for the patient, a steady hand, patience, good eyes and the ability to work hard. If you combine these virtues with the proper electrology education and the assistance of a good instructor, your career as professional electrologists will be a successful one.

My Best Wishes,

Fino Gior

Contents

Chapter 1 Hair Removal, Past And Present

LEARNING OBJECTIVES   Successful mastery of the material in this chapter will be indicated when you can:

1. Briefly describe the hair removal methods used in ancient times.
2. Indicate the types of current used for electrolysis, thermolysis, and blend treatments.
3. List five controversial methods of hair removal and be able to discuss their areas of dispute.
4. Describe the procedure for at least four methods of temporary hair removal.

INTRODUCTION   Unwanted hair has presented problems to individuals for thousands of years. As an electrology student today, you will study early methods of hair removal, and then learn the terminology of current electrology techniques and equipment.

When performed by a competent electrologist, the permanent method of hair removal becomes the *most practical* as well as the *most economical* solution to the problem of superfluous hair.

HISTORICAL METHODS   One of the earliest methods of hair removal known was the use of an abrasive, such as pumice stone, to wear away the hair. Excavations of early Egyptian tombs have revealed abrasives used for this purpose. Ancient Greek and Roman women were known to remove most of their body hair by abrasion. The American Indian sharpened stones and sea shells and then rubbed off and plucked out hair. Abrasives continue to be a method of removing unwanted hair today.

History also records chemical means of removing excess hair. The ancient Turkish people, for example, used rusma, a combination of yellow sulfide of arsenic, quicklime, and rose water, as a crude depilatory. Most chemical depilatories used today also have an alkaline pH to assist in the decomposition of the hair.

CURRENT METHODS   Let us now examine the current categories of hair removal. They are:

1. **Permanent** methods that destroy the hair **papilla,** preventing any further hair growth.
2. **Experimental** methods that are still under development or disputed, including **drugs.**
3. **Temporary** methods that are repeated as the hair regrows.

Permanent Methods

The first effective technique of permanent hair removal invented was electrolysis. The technique was devised by an ophthalmologist, Charles E. Michel of St. Louis, Missouri, in 1875. Dr. Michel had tried for many years to solve the problem of ingrown eyelashes, which caused severe irritations.

Trying a new technique to solve the problem, Michel attached a very fine conductor wire to a dry cell battery. He then attached the wire to a surgical needle and inserted it into the follicle of the eyelash. After the treatment the hair did not regrow and history was made.

The electrolysis treatment devised by Dr. Michel used a *galvanic* or direct current. The electricity chemically decomposed the **dermal papilla** of the hair follicle.

The direct current process was time-consuming and tedious. In 1916. Professor Paul Kree developed a **multiple galvanic machine.** This allowed the electrologist to insert up to 10 needles in time sequence instead of spending several minutes on each hair. (Multiple galvanic technique will be discussed in Chapter 3.)

In 1924, Dr. H. Brodier of Paris developed **thermolysis** *(thur MOL i sis)*, a method of hair removal using high frequency or alternating current. This method created heat to destroy the papilla, and soon became popular because it was a much faster technique.

In 1945, Henri St. Pierre and Arthur Hinkel successfully blended galvanic current with a high frequency current of low intensity. The currents ran simultaneously through a single tapered needle. This blend method was devised to destroy the dermal papilla and **germinative** *(jur MI nah tiv)* cells by decomposition much faster than galvanic current used alone.

OTHER MODERN HAIR REMOVAL METHODS

X Ray

Many experimental devices have been explored. This includes the X ray, which was used in hair removal for several years. Use of the X ray proved to be disastrous as it not only removed the hair, but also damaged tissue in the area of the body being treated. X ray use resulted in illness and even death.

Photoepilation

The **photoepilation** *(FOH toh ep i LAY shun)* device utilized a blue-green light, which was channeled into the hair follicle by fiber optics. The manufacturers of the device claimed that the light would react with the color red in the blood. This would stop the blood supply so that there would be no further hair growth.

In 1974, a lawsuit challenged these claims and the device was taken off the market.

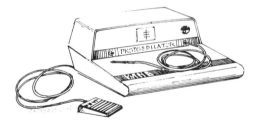

The Photoepilator was once thought to stop hair growth.

Laser

In the 1980s the first laser device was introduced into the permanent hair removal profession. It was an *argon laser* that never caught hold because it never proved to be effective, it was very costly and the equipment was very large.

A laser device may contain a gas or mineral such as carbon or ruby crystal and when stimulated with the proper electric current the atoms will focus a cohesive light beam that will react with anything black.

The beam will vaporize the black hair, but will not have any effect on blond, gray or vellus hair. The theory is that if there is enough of the pigment melanin in the follicle itself there would be permanent follicle destruction. Unfortunately there is not enough melanin in the hair follicle to cause substantial amounts of permanent tissue destruction.

This is why, in my opinion, the FDA Medical Device Division gave clearance for a few of these devices to advertise, "Permanent Reduction." There is a little destruction but not enough to call it Permanent.

To date the laser has not proved itself to be as sufficiently effective as needle type electrology. In most cases that I have examined there was no permanent hair removal at all.

Electronic Tweezer

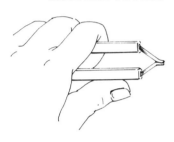

In 1975, a new device was introduced for the removal of superfluous hair. This device claimed to offer painless hair removal by means of radio frequency. The **electronic tweezer** transmits radio frequency (r.f.) energy down the hair shaft into the follicle area. Claims state that the papilla is thus dehydrated and eventually destroyed.

The radio frequency is applied to the hair by a tweezer. When the tweezer is energized, r.f. energy is transmitted through the moist area of the hair bulb and papilla, causing it to coagulate. In theory, very little of the radio frequency is lost along the shaft of the hair because of the hair-to-air-to-skin connection in the follicle.

Investigation, however, has lead to the conclusion that the apparatus is not effective as a permanent hair removal device. The United States Food and Drug Administration issued an opinion that electronic tweezers cannot advertise as a method of permanent hair removal. The Federal Trade Commission also stated that the manufacturers of these devices may not advertise them for permanent hair removal.

Drugs

Medical researchers are now experimenting with the use of drugs to cure unwanted hair. The concept is to intercept the hormone factors which cause hair growth. These drugs are commonly called anti-androgen or androgen blocs.

Cimetidine, *(si MET i deen)*, also known as **Tagamet,** *(TAG ah met)* is a drug used in the treatment of ulcers. This drug has shown some effectiveness as an anti-androgen. Cimetidine has the possible side effects of diarrhea, dizziness, muscle pain, rash, and kidney disease. There is speculation that cimetidine could be a carcinogen or cause blood and cardiac abnormalities.

Spironolactone *(speye ROH no LAK tohn)*, also known as **Aldactone** *(al DAK tohn)*, is a diuretic. Side effects are interference with the menstrual cycle and possible breast cancer.

17-A-methyl-B-testosterone *(17-ay-METH-il-B-tes* **TOS** *te rohn)* and **Cyproterone** *(seye PROH ter ohn)* are two other experimental drugs. Cyproterone has become more popular in European countries where restrictions are not as rigid as in the United States.

None of these drugs have been approved by the Food and Drug Administration as treatments for **hirsutism** *(HER soot izm)* because of the side effects, and the difficulty of localizing reactions to the portion of the body being treated.

The **hirsute** *(HER soot)* female, whose problem is traced to an **adrenal** *(a DREE nal)* or **ovarian** *(oh VAIR i an)* cause, may be treated with **prednisone** *(PRED ni sohn)* or **dexamethosone.** Women may also be treated with "the pill," although few experience a change in their excess hair problems. In some cases their problem was stabilized, but existing hair does not fall out. Many have grown even more hair within a three month period.

Home Methods

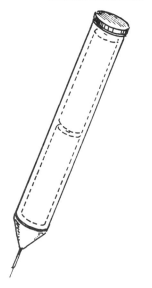

Home electrolysis device.

Home electrolysis devices are also available. Manufacturers claim that anyone can purchase these devices, follow the instructions, and permanently and safely remove hair. The consumer is interested in what appears to be a much less expensive approach to hair removal. In some areas, however, these devices are not legal.

The Food and Drug Administration's *Consumer's Report* warns, "Consumers should be particularly careful about using any of the home electrolysis devices... Considerable skill and dexterity is required to perform electrolysis properly, and most people would probably be better off going to an expert instead of trying it themselves."

The British Medical Association Dermatologist's Group Committee declared home devices unsafe when several women were scarred trying to manipulate the needle in their skin.

Most manufacturers admit that some portions of the body cannot be treated easily or even at all. A person's back, for instance, cannot be reached. Also there are other problems of proper lighting, magnification of the area to be treated, and proper needle insertion. The person attempting home treatment must, at times, work in reverse using a mirror.

Scarring can result from an unsteady hand or from inserting the needle for too long.

Another area of concern is the high risk of infection with these devices. Without proper sterilization of the needle, infection is a very real possibility.

Most users complain that home devices require too much time as the needle has to stay in the hair follicle for too long (approximately 45 seconds per hair when the battery is fresh, and longer as the battery ages). The devices are also limited as to needle size. In most cases, the size needle is too wide for fine hair follicles.

TEMPORARY METHODS
Shaving

Shaving is the most popular of all methods of hair removal. Shaving cream and a razor blade is the most popular technique used today. The electric razor is another shaving option. Both are relatively safe. Cuts and rashes are rare and usually superficial. There have been claims that shaving makes the hair grow faster and thicker, but this is *not* true. The area shaved *seems* thicker because the thicker portion of the hair is left behind and held rigid by the follicle.

Tweezing

Tweezing is a method in which a hair is manually pulled from the follicle. A tweezer is most commonly used. Since this method can only remove one hair at a time, only a small area can be treated. Eyebrows, the chin, and the upper lip are the areas most commonly treated this way.

Waxing

Waxing is done on larger body areas or where more hair exists, such as the legs, the arms, or even the back. A depilatory wax is heated and applied in strips usually 3 inches wide by 6 inches long. A piece of sterile muslin is then placed over the wax. As the wax cools and hardens, it surrounds and adheres to the hair and the muslin. The muslin is pulled away from the skin in the opposite direction of the hair growth, pulling the hair out.

REMOVING UNWANTED
HAIR FROM THE LEGS
WITH SOFT WAX
Step-By-Step Procedure

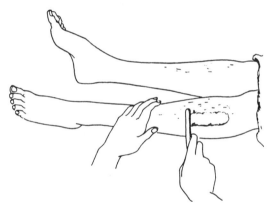

While holding the spatula at a 45⁰ angle, apply a thin film of wax to the area being treated. Draw the spatula in the direction of the hair growth.

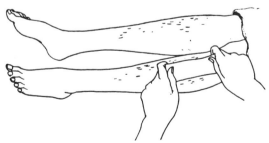

Stretch the muslin strip directly over the wax application. Allow enough free edge of the fabric for the hand to grasp for removal.

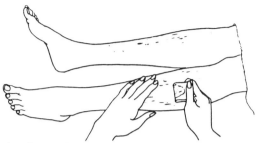

Grasp the free edge of the strip tightly with one hand while holding the other hand against the skin to hold the skin taut. Quickly pull the strip in the opposite direction of the hair growth. Be sure the hand pulling the strip remains close to the skin. The area covered by the strip should be clean and free of hair.

Waxing is faster than tweezing. Most areas will remain clean and smooth for several weeks. There are some disadvantages, however. The hair does grow back and for some patients under 35 it will grow back even thicker in diameter. Lee McCarthy, M.D., states in *Diagnosis and Treatment of Diseases of the Hair,* "Although at first scarcely perceptible, it is undoubtedly true that in the long run continuously repeated epilations (tweezing) cause the hair to regrow a little more quickly, a little larger in diameter, and stronger."

Ingrown hairs can be another drawback of waxing. This happens when the hair is pulled apart inside the hair follicle. Instead of growing up and out of the follicle, the hair curls under the skin causing a cyst-like projection. There is also the possibility of the wax being heated to a temperature high enough to cause burns, especially in sensitive areas.

Another problem with waxing is that the hair must be long enough for the procedure to be successful. This means the patient must allow the hair to grow many weeks before it can be waxed.

Chemical Depilatories

Chemical depilatories are solvents that break down the hair. They are available as pastes, creams, and powders that are mixed with water. Many of these products make claims of eventual permanent removal, but no scientific evidence has ever been established to prove them.

The procedure is relatively easy. The consumer applies the chemical depilatory directly to the area where hair removal is desired and times the process according to the manufacturer's instructions, usually 5 to 10 minutes. The chemical is then rinsed off with warm water, the area is gently patted dry, and soothing cream or lotion is applied.

A sensitivity test should be taken by applying the product to a small area as directed. If at the end of the required time there are no signs of redness or swelling, the depilatory may be used safely. Chemical depilatories should not be used around the eyes and pubic region.

Abrasives   As we discussed earlier, abrasives are the oldest method of temporary hair removal. The pumice stone is used to this day. All abrasive methods entail a rubbing back and forth until the hair is worn away. This procedure causes enough friction to cause irritation, and on sensitive skins may cause burns. A cool soothing lotion should be applied after treatment.

Bleaching   Hair lightening methods do not remove hair, but they do make it less noticeable. The time required to lighten the hair depends on how dark and how thick the hairs are. Fine **lanugo** *(lah NOO goh)* hair reacts faster to lighteners than does dark terminal hair.

Most bleaching products are sold commercially. They usually consist of a powder and a cream that must be mixed before it is applied to the hair. 15 to 50 minutes is required, depending on the thickness of the hair, before it will be light enough. The area must be tested for sensitivity before treatment.

QUESTIONS FOR
REVIEW:

1. What methods were used in ancient times for the removal of unwanted hair.
2. What type of current is used for electrolysis? For thermolysis? For blend treatments?
3. What are five controversial methods of hair removal? Why are each of the methods controversial?
4. What is the procedure for temporary hair removal by shaving? By tweezing? How are waxes and chemical depilatories applied? How does an abrasive temporarily remove hair?

Chapter 2 Basic Electricity

Successful mastery of the material in this chapter will be indicated when you can:

1. Name five sources of electricity.
2. List the types of electricity available.
3. List the three modalities for electrology, and briefly
   describe how each works.
4. Define the primary terms used to describe electrology
   equipment.
5. List eight safety precautions for the electrologist.

INTRODUCTION Electrology uses electrical energy to cause the permanent
destruction of the hair papilla. The professional technician must
study electricity in order to understand the effects of treatment
and to evaluate equipment. A well educated electrologist will
easily recognize effective apparatus and avoid poor investments
in faulty equipment.

ELECTRICITY In about 600 B.C., Thales, a Greek philosopher, rubbed a
piece of amber fossil with fur. Lightweight objects such as
feathers attached themselves to the amber. In a later era, Sir
William Gilbert, physician to Queen Elizabeth I, observed that
many substances behaved like amber after being rubbed. He
said the substances became **electrified,** from the Greek word
"electron," for amber. And so began the study of electricity,
which continues to this very day.

The exact nature of electricity is not understood. We do know
that it has many sources such as friction, magnetism, heat,
chemical, and atomic reactions.

TYPES OF ELECTRICITY **Electricity** is the flow of electrons (negatively charged particles) along a conductor. Two types of electricity are used,
namely:

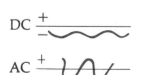

1. **Direct current** (DC) is a constant and even-flowing current,
   traveling in one direction.
2. **Alternating current** (AC) is a rapid and interrupted current,
   flowing first in one direction and then in the opposite direction.

If necessary, one type of current can be changed to the other by means of a **converter** or **rectifier.**

A **converter** is an apparatus used to convert direct current into alternating current. A **rectifier** is used to change an alternating current into a direct current.

Electrical Terminology

The following are definitions of some common electrical terms:

Conductor: A conductor is a substance which readily transmits electrical current. Most metals (especially copper), water solutions of acid or salt, and the human body, are good conductors. Surgical stainless steel needles are the most frequently utilized conductors in electrology treatment.

Nonconductor: A nonconductor, or **insulator,** is a substance that resists the passage of an electrical current. Rubber, plastic, glass, dry wood, and even hair itself are insulators of electricity.

Circuit: The circuit of electricity is the entire path traveled by the current, from its generating source through conductors (for example, machine, needle holder, needle, human body), and back to its original source.

Fuse: A fuse is a safety device which prevents the overheating of electrical wires. Overheating can occur when too many machines or appliances are plugged into one source. If the circuit is overloaded, the fuse will cut the electrical current. To reestablish the circuit:

1. Disconnect the apparatus.
2. Use a new fuse with the proper rating.
3. Stand on a dry surface and keep hands dry to prevent shock.
4. Replace fuse and reconnect apparatus.
5. Have the equipment checked for the cause of the short.

Circuit breaker: A circuit breaker is a switch used in place of a fuse. The circuit breaker automatically breaks the current when it is overloaded. Power is restored by flicking the switch to On, although the cause for the power overload must first be eliminated.

Electrical Measurements

Electrical measurements are expressed in terms of the following units:

Volt: the unit of electrical pressure.
Ampere: the unit of electrical strength.
Ohm: the unit of electrical resistance.
Watt: the unit of power, or amperes times volts.

An electrical current flows through a conductor when the pressure is sufficient to overcome the resistance the wire offers to the current's passage. According to Ohm's law, the strength of a current (amperage) equals the pressure (voltage) divided by the resistance (ohm).

$$A = \frac{V}{O}$$

If we increase the voltage applied to the circuit, the electron flow becomes stronger. Reducing the voltage makes the current weaker.

If we leave the voltage the same, increasing the resistance will make the current weaker. Reducing the resistance will naturally allow more current to flow.

Instead of the ampere which is too strong, the **milliampere** *(MIL i AM peer)*, one-thousandth of an ampere, is the unit of measure used in electrology treatments. The **milliamperemeter** *(MIL i am PEER mee tur)* is an instrument for measuring the rate of flow of an electric current.

MODALITIES OF ELECTROLOGY

There are three modalities, or modes, of electricity that are used in electrology. They are:

Electrolysis
Thermolysis
Blend (a combination of Electrolysis and Thermolysis)

Electrolysis

Electrolysis is the use of direct current to change the chemical composition of the papilla. The current used by Dr. Michel for his battery-operated apparatus was direct current. **Direct current** (DC) is a constant flow of electrons in one direction through a conductor. Direct current is also known as **galvanic current.**

Iontophoresis. When using galvanic current, there are two poles; a negative pole (-), and a positive pole (+). These **polarities** *(poh LAR i teez)* can cause what is termed **iontophoresis** *(i ON to fo REE sis)*. Iontophoresis is a method of introducing water soluble products into the skin.

Test for Polarity. The electrologist should know which is the positive and which is the negative pole. Most galvanic machines have a polarity indicator. If necessary, polarity can be tested as follows:

1. Separate the tips of the two conducting cords and immerse them in a glass of salt water. Turn up the current of the milliamperemeter. As the water breaks down, more bubbles will gather to the negative pole then to the positive.
2. Place the tips of the two conducting cords on moistened litmus paper. Red litmus will turn blue under the negative pole, and blue litmus will turn red under the positive pole.

NOTE: *It is the negative pole that produces the decomposition of the hair follicle tissue.*

Anaphoresis. Anaphoresis *(AN ah fo REE sis)* is the use of the negative pole or cathode to produce an alkaline effect on the skin. Anaphoresis increases blood supply, softens skin, and stimulates nerves. The negative pole is used as the treatment pole in all modalities of permanent hair removal.

Cataphoresis. Cataphoresis *(KAT ah fo REE sis)* is the use of the positive pole or anode to produce an acid effect on the skin. Cataphoresis closes follicles, decreases redness, and brings the skin back to its proper pH after electrolysis treatment.

Thermolysis   Thermolysis is the use of alternating current, usually in the form of high frequency or radio waves. This mode of electrology uses heat produced by friction to achieve permanent hair removal.

Alternating current oscillates between 10 and 15,000 cycles per second. Radio frequencies have been internationally categorized as VHF (Very High Frequency) and UHF (Ultra High Frequency). VHF has a range of 30 to 300 megahertz and UHF has a range of 300 to 30,000 megahertz. Megahertz is a unit of frequency equal to one million cycles per second.

High frequency is used by the majority of electrologists today.

FCC Law. The Federal Communications Commission (FCC) has set aside three frequencies for electrology equipment. They are 13.56, 27.12, and 40.68 **megahertz** *(MEG a hurts)*. The use of any other frequency is against Federal Law.

FCC approval merely indicates that the apparatus is operating within lawful frequencies. *It does not indicate government approval, sanction, or effectiveness.*

Blend   The blend modality of electrolysis combines direct and alternating currents. The currents may be used together or sequentially.

TERMINOLOGY FOR ELECTROLOGY EQUIPMENT   Some terms for common electrology equipment are defined as follows:

Jack: A jack is a fitting device found on the end of an electrical cord or needle holder. It is inserted into the receptacle on the machine.

Plug: The plug is the part of an electrical cord that connects the machine to the electrical outlet. The jack and the plug complete the circuit.

Electrode *(i LEK trohd):* An electrode is the positive or negative terminal of an electrical source.

Polarity changer: A polarity changer alters the direction of electrical current.

Transformer *(trans FDR mer):* A transformer is used with alternating currents to either step up (increase) or step down (decrease) alternating voltage.

Rectifier *(REK ti feye er):* A rectifier is a device used to change alternating current into direct current.

Converter *(kon VUR ter):* A converter is a device used to change direct current into alternating current.

Filter *(FIL ter):* A filter alters the wave length of direct current. It utilizes a condenser, or capacitor, to store electrical energy.

Oscillator *(OS i LAY tor):* An oscillator is a device used to produce higher frequency alternating currents. Oscillators produce rapid changes in polarity, measured in **megahertz,** (millions of oscillations per second).

Rheostat *(REE o stat):* The rheostat regulates the strength of a current. It is also known as the **intensity control.**

SAFETY PRACTICES
IN ELECTRICITY

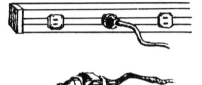

Use only one plug to each outlet. Overloading may cause fuse to blow out.

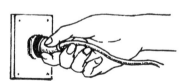

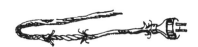

To disconnect current, remove plug without pulling cord. Never pull on cord as the wires may become loosened, and may cause a short circuit.

Examine cords regularly. Repair or replace worn cords to prevent short circuit, shock or fire.

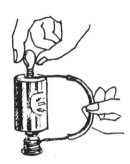

WARNING: Keep a flashlight at top of steps, so you won't stumble down a dark stairway. Using your flashlight, open fuse box and examine each fuse to locate "dead" one. When you replace a burned-out fuse, touch only its rim. Never put a coin in the fuse box instead of a fuse.

Be sure to have some good fuses on hand. To test a fuse, use a flashlight battery, and bulb (or the bulb assembly), and a piece of wire—as shown at left. If fuse is good, bulb will light.

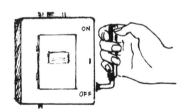

In an emergency, turn off main switch, as illustrated, to shut off electricity.

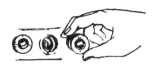

When replacing a blown-out fuse, make sure to:

1. Use new fuse with proper rating.
2. Stand on a dry surface.
3. Keep hands dry.

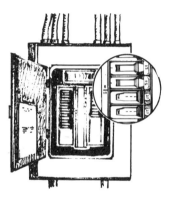

Circuit breakers are now the most commonly used device for protecting electrical circuits. When there is an overload condition, the switch or breaker simply moves automatically from the "on" to the "off" position. To reset, first switch off or unplug whatever appliances were being used on the circuit. Open the door of the circuit breaker panel to see which of the breakers has moved to the "off" position. Keep in mind that the breaker switch does not always move all the way to the "off" position, but slightly away from the "on." To re-establish power, move the breaker switch all the way to the "off" position then snap it back to the "on" position. Close the circuit breaker door. Resume the use of the appliance. If the circuit breaker again shuts off power, then it is likely that there is a short in the appliance being used, or the circuit is overloaded with too many appliances.

SAFETY PRECAUTIONS

1. Read instructions before using any electrical equipment.
2. Disconnect equipment when you are finished using it.
3. Inspect all electrical equipment frequently.
4. Keep all wires, plugs, and equipment in good condition.
5. Avoid getting electrical equipment or cords wet.
6. Sanitize all electrodes properly.
7. When using electrical equipment, protect the patient at all times.
8. Do not touch any metal while using electrical equipment.
9. Do not handle electrical equipment with wet hands.
10. Do not allow patient to touch any metal surfaces while being treated with electrical equipment.
11. Do not attempt to clean the area around an electric outlet when equipment is connected.

QUESTIONS FOR REWIEW

1. What are the sources of electricity?
2. What are the types of electricity available?
3. What are the three modalities for electrology?
4. What are the primary parts of electrology equipment?
5. What are eight safety precautions for the electrologist to follow?

Chapter 3 Chemistry for Electrologists

INTRODUCTION Chemistry *(KEM is tree)* is important to the student electrologist. A basic knowledge of this science is essential in order to understand various products that are used in electrology treatments. The reactions of these preparations on the skin before and after treatment are of concern.

New products are constantly being developed. It is important that the professional understand these products and learn how to use them so that the patient will receive the maximum benefit.

The galvanic modality of electrolysis involves a chemical reaction in the follicle, making the study of chemistry fundamental for any professional electrologist.

CHEMISTRY DEFINED Chemistry is the study of the composition, structure, and properties of matter, and the capacity of matter to change under different conditions.

Organic Chemistry

Organic chemistry *(or GAH nik KEM is tree)* is the study of all substances which are carbon-based and which are generally thought of as living or once living matter. These substances can be dissolved by organic **solvents,** *(SOL vents)* such as **alcohol** *(AL ko hawl)* and **benzene** *(BEN zeen).* They are not **soluble** *(SOL yoo bel)* in water. Most organic substances will burn, but are slow in their chemical reactions.

Examples of organic substances are skin, hair, oil, soap, detergents, plastics, and **antibiotics** *(an ti beye OT iks).*

Inorganic Chemistry

Inorganic chemistry *(in or GAN ik KEM is tree)* is the study of all substances that are not carbon-based and are not living, including the elements.

Inorganic substances are quick in their chemical reactions. Examples of inorganic substances are water, air, needles, iron, lead and iodine. Electrology needles, which are made of steel, are inorganic.

MATTER

Matter *(MAT er)* is defined as anything that occupies space and has weight. Matter exists in three forms: solids, liquids, and gases.

Look around the classroom and note what you see: hair, people, desks, chairs, walls. These items are matter in the solid state.

In the electrology office, you see water, lotions, and **antiseptics** *(an ti SEP tiks).* These are examples of matter in the liquid state. Air is matter in the **gaseous** *(GAS ee us)* state.

Matter exists in an **infinite** *(IN fih nit)* variety. This is due to the atomic structure of matter, which permits the elements to join in countless combinations. When we talk about the *chemical activity* of an element, we refer to its ability to combine with other elements. For example, **hydrogen** *(HEYE dro jen)* is a very active element and readily combines with other elements, while neon is completely inactive and does not combine with other elements.

Atoms

An **atom** *(AT om)* is the smallest part of an *element* that possesses the characteristics of that element. Therefore, an atom of hydrogen has the properties of hydrogen. Should the atom be split, this would no longer be true.

Molecules

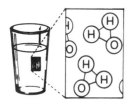

A **molecule** *(MOL eh kyool)* is the smallest particle of an **element** *(EL e ment)* or **compound** *(KOM pound)* that possesses all the properties of the element or compound. If the molecule is of an element, the atoms are all the same. If it is of a compound (a union of separate elements), the atoms are different. For example, a molecule of hydrogen contains two or more atoms of hydrogen, but a molecule of water is composed of two atoms of hydrogen and one atom of oxygen (H_2O).

ELEMENTS, COMPOUNDS, AND MIXTURES

Elements. An element, as we know, is the simplest form of matter. It cannot be broken down into a simpler chemical substance. There are now 105 known elements; some of the more common are iron, sulphur, oxygen, zinc, and silver.

Each element has a letter symbol:

Iron . . . . Fe

Sulphur . . . . S

Oxygen . . . . O

Zinc . . . . Zn

Silver . . . . Ag

All symbols can be obtained by referring to a chart of elements called the Periodic Table.

Compounds. As mentioned above, when two or more elements unite chemically, they form a compound. In this process each element loses its individual properties and the new compound develops its own characteristics. For example, iron oxide (rust) has different properties from the two elements of which it is composed: iron and oxygen. The new substance, which is a compound, cannot be altered by mechanical means, it can only be changed by chemical methods.

ELEMENTS AND COMPOUNDS

Matter
Solids
Gases
Liquids

TYPES AND DEFINITION	SMALLEST PARTICLE
ELEMENTS	*ATOM*
Simplest Form of Matter	*(Cannot be broken down by simple chemical reactions.) About 100 different kinds.*
COMPOUNDS	
Formed by Combination of Elements.	*MOLECULE*
	(Consists of 2 or more atoms chemically combined.) Unlimited kinds possible.

ELEMENTS FOUND IN SKIN OR HAIR	COMPOUNDS USED ON SKIN OR HAIR
CARBON	*WATER*
NITROGEN	*HYDROGEN PEROXIDE*
OXYGEN	*AMMONIUM THIOGLYCOLATE*
SULFUR	*ALCOHOL*
HYDROGEN	*ALKALIS*
PHOSPHORUS	

Compounds are divided into many classes. Four that are common in electrology are:

1. **Oxides** *(OK seyeds)* are compounds consisting of any element combined with oxygen. For example, one part carbon and two parts oxygen equal **carbon dioxide** *(KAHR bon deye OK seyed)*, which might be recognized as dry ice. Or, one part carbon and one part oxygen equal carbon monoxide better known as the poisonous exhaust of an automobile. Oxides are commonly used as pigment.

2. **Acids** are compounds of hydrogen, a nonmetal such as **nitrogen** *(NEYE troh jen)* and sometimes, oxygen. For example, hydrogen + **chlorine** *(KLOHR een)* (Cl) = **hydrochloric acid** *(HEYE droh KLOHR ik AS id)* (HCl), which forms at the positive pole in galvanic electrolysis. This is the acid which breaks down steel needles and leaves black spots on the skin. Acids turn blue **litmus** *(LIT muhs)* paper red, providing a quick way to test a compound. Most aftertreatment lotions and creams contain acids to soothe the skin.

3. **Bases,** also known as **alkalies** *(AL kah leyes)*, are compounds of hydrogen, a metal, and oxygen. For example, sodium + hydrogen = **sodium hydroxide** *(SOH dee um hy DRAHKS yd)*, (NaOH), which is used in the process of galvanic electrolysis.

4. **Salts** are chemical compounds which are formed along with water when an acid and a base react together. Two common salts and their formulas are **sodium chloride** *(SOH dee um KLOHR eyd)* table salt, (NaCl), which contains sodium and chloride (it is this salt solution which is found in the skin and is responsible for galvanic electrology); and **magnesium sulfate** *(mag NEE zee um SUL fayt)*, Epsom salts, $MgSo_4$, which contains magnesium, sulphur, hydrogen and oxygen.

Mixtures. A mixture *(MIKS chur)* is a substance that is made up of two elements, combined physically rather than chemically. The ingredients in a mixture do not change their properties, but retain their individual characteristics. For example, concrete is composed of sand, gravel and cement. While concrete is a mixture having its own functions, its ingredients never lose their characteristics. Sand remains sand, gravel is still gravel, and cement, cement.

CHANGES IN MATTER

Matter may be changed in two ways: physical or chemical.

Physical Changes

Physical change refers to the altering of the properties of matter without forming any new substance. For example, ice, a solid, melts at a certain temperature and becomes water, a liquid. Yet water freezes at a certain temperature and becomes a solid. There is no change in the nature of the water, merely a change in its form. A physical change occurs during thermolysis treatment.

PROPERTIES OF COMMON ELEMENTS, COMPOUNDS, AND MIXTURES

Knowledge of the properties of some of the most common elements, compounds and mixtures can be helpful to the electrologist in understanding why certain reactions occur.

Oxygen

Oxygen (O) is the most abundant element found both free and in compounds. It composes about half of the earth's crust, half of the rock, one-fifth of the air, and 90% of the water. It is a colorless, odorless, tasteless, gaseous substance, combining with most other elements to form an infinite variety of compounds, called oxides. One of the chief characteristics of this element is its ability to support combustion.

Hydrogen

Hydrogen (H) is a colorless, odorless, tasteless gas, and is the lightest element known. It is inflammable and explosive when mixed with air. It is found in chemical combination with oxygen in water, and with other elements in acids, bases and organic substances like wood, meat, fish, sugar and butter.

Air

Air is the gaseous mixture which makes up the earth's atmosphere. It is odorless, colorless, and generally consists of about one part by volume of oxygen and four parts of nitrogen. It also contains a small amount of carbon dioxide, **ammonia** *(ah MOHN yah)*, and organic matter, which are all essential to plant and animal life.

Hydrogen Peroxide

Hydrogen peroxide *(HEYE droh jen peh ROK seyd)*, (H_2O_2) is a compound of hydrogen and oxygen. It is a colorless liquid with a characteristic odor and slightly acid taste. A 10 volume solution of hydrogen peroxide possesses antiseptic qualities.

Nitrogen

Nitrogen (N) is a colorless, gaseous element found free in the air. It constitutes part of the atmosphere, forming about four-fifths of the air, and is necessary to life because it dilutes the oxygen. It is found chiefly in the form of ammonia and **nitrates** *(NEYE trayts)*

ACIDITY AND ALKALINITY (pH SCALE)

To an electrologist, pH is a value used to indicate the **acidity** *(ah SID i tee)* or **alkalinity** *(al kah LIN i tee)* of water-based solutions. This pH value can be measured through the use of meters and indicators. The acidity or alkalinity of a cosmetic product is important to the electrologist because it influences how the product will affect the skin.

The pH scale goes from 0.0 to 14.0. The neutral point is 7.0. Each increase of 1 indicates a tenfold increase of alkalinity and a tenfold decrease of acidity.

Acidity

Anything below 7.0 is acid. The lower the pH, the greater the degree of acidity.

Alkalinity

Anything from 7.0 to 14.0 is alkaline. The higher the pH, the greater the degree of alkalinity.

Neutrality

Although the precise neutral point on the pH scale is 7.0, the neutral range is considered to extend from 6.5 to 7.5.

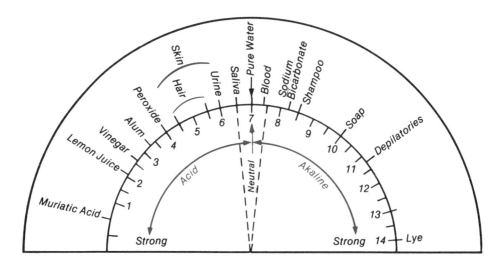

Average pH Values

The pH a product can usually be tested by the use of **indicator papers.** When the indicator papers are dipped in a substance that is acid, they will turn pink or orange. If the substance is alkaline, the papers will turn green or blue. This procedure should be used when testing polarity, for the galvanic or blend methods.

The pH of the skin ranges from 4.5 to 6.0, and is most often referred to as 5.5. It is generally believed that unless a cosmetic has a pH of 5.5 it is not compatible with the skin. Actually, many products would not be as effective if they had a reading of 5.5. For example, a cleanser formulated with a pH of 7.0, which is neutral, (the same as pure water) will cleanse the skin better than a cleanser with a pH a 5.5. A **moisturizer** *(MOIS chu reyez er)* that is slightly alkaline will have a softening effect on the skin. This makes it easier for the skin to absorb the beneficial ingredients in the moisturizer.

CHEMISTRY OF WATER

Water (H_2O) is the most abundant of all substances, composing about 75% of the earth's surface, and about 65% of the human body. It is the universal solvent. **Demineralized** *(de MIN er al eyezd)* or distilled water is used as a nonconductor of electricity. Water containing certain mineral substances is an excellent conductor of electricity.

Water is necessary for both galvanic and thermolysis electrology. It is moisture that heats to a degree sufficient enough to destroy tissue in thermolysis. It is salt water in tissue that causes the chemical reaction in the galvanic method.

Water serves many useful purposes in the office. Its main use for the electrologist is in washing before and after giving a treatment. Only water of known purity is fit for drinking purposes. Suspended or dissolved impurities in water make it unsatisfactory for cleaning objects and for use in electrology treatment.

Sterilization of Water

In most cases distilled or filtered water is used in the office for machines that require water. Boiling water at a temperature of 212° F (100° C), will destroy most microbic life.

CHEMISTRY AS APPLIED TO COSMETICS

Electrologists will be better equipped to serve the public if they have an understanding of the chemical composition, preparation and uses of before and after treatment cosmetics that are intended to cleanse, protect, and sanitize the treatment area.

Cosmetics may be classified according to their physical and chemical nature and the characteristics by which they are recognized. The object in classifying cosmetics is to assist in their identification.

Physical and Chemical Classifications of Pharmaceutical Preparations

The following are six classifications of **pharmaceutical** *(fahr mah SOO ti kahl)* preparations the electrologist should be familiar with:

1. Powders
2. Solutions
3. Suspensions
4. Emulsions
5. Ointments
6. Pastes

Powders. A **powder** is a uniform mixture of insoluble substances (inorganic, organic and **colloidal** *(ko LOY dahl)* which have been properly blended, perfumed and/or tinted to produce a preparation which is free from coarse or gritty particles.

In the process of making powders, mixing and shifting processes are employed.

Solutions. A **solution** is a preparation made by dissolving a solid, liquid or gaseous substance in another substance, usually liquid.

A **solute** *(SOL yoot)* is a substance dissolved in a solution.

A **solvent** *(SOL vent)* is a liquid used to dissolve a solute.

Solutions are clear and are permanent mixtures of solutes and solvents which do not separate on standing. Since a good solution is clear and transparent, **filtration** *(fil TRAY shun)* is often necessary, particularly if the solution is cloudy.

Solutions are easily prepared by dissolving and stirring a powdered solute in a warm solvent. The solute may be separated from the solvent by the application of heat which evaporates the solvent.

Water is known as the **universal solvent.** This means it is capable of dissolving more substances than any other solvent. Grain alcohol and **glycerine** *(GLIS eh rin)* are frequently used as solvents. Water, glycerine and alcohol readily mix with each other which makes them **miscible** *(MIS ih bel)*. On the other hand, water and oil do not mix with each other; they are **immiscible** *(i MIS is bel)*. In general, inorganic solvents dissolve inorganic substances and organic solvents dissolve organic substances.

The solute may be either a solid, liquid or gas. For example, boric acid solution is made by dissolving a solid in a liquid; glycerine and rose water is a mixture of two miscible liquids; ammonia water is a solution of a gas in water.

Solutions containing **volatile** *(VOL ah til)* substances, such as ammonia and alcohol, should be stored in a cool place; otherwise, the volatile substance will evaporate.

There are various kinds of solutions:

A **dilute solution** contains a small quantity of solute in proportion to the quantity of solvent.

A **concentrated solution** contains a large quantity of solute in proportion to the quantity of solvent.

A **saturated** *(S ACH u rayt ed) solution* will not dissolve or take up more of the solute than it already holds at a given temperature.

Suspensions. Suspensions *(su SPEN shuns)* are temporary mixtures of **insoluble** *(in SOL yoo bel)* powders in liquid. Since the particles have a tendency to separate on standing, a thorough shaking is required before using. A suspension should not be filtered. Some skin lotions are actually suspensions. [Example: **calamine** *(KAL ah meyen)* lotion.]

Suspensions are made by first mixing the powders, then adding a small amount of liquid to form a smooth paste, and finally adding the balance of the liquid.

Emulsions. Emulsions *(i MUL shuns)* (creams) are permanent mixtures of two or more immiscible substances (like oil and water) which are united with the aid of a binder or **emulsifier** *(i MUL si feye er)*. Emulsions are usually milky white in appearance. If a suitable emulsifier and the proper technique are employed, the resulting emulsion will be stable. A stable emulsion can hold as much as 90% water. Depending on the amount of water and wax present, the cream may be either liquid or semisolid in character. The amount of emulsifier used depends on its efficiency and the amount of water or oil to be emulsified.

Emulsions are prepared by hand or with the aid of a grinding and cutting machine, called a colloidal mill. In the process of preparing the emulsion, the emulsifier forms a protective film around the **microscopic** *(meye kro SKOP ik)*, **globules** *(GLOB yools)* of either the oil or the water. The smaller the globules, the thicker and more stable the emulsion will be.

Emulsions are used to overcome the difficulties of applying substances which are insoluble in water to the skin. For example, oils are required to condition the **epidermis** *(ep i DUR mis)* of the skin, either as a special preparation (antiseptic) or as a soothing agent. If an emulsifier is present, it will coat the droplets of oil as they are formed. This stabilizes the oils and forms an emulsion. There are two types of emulsions, oil-in-water (O/W) and water-in-oil (W/O). Oil-in-water emulsions are made of oil droplets dispersed in a watery base and water-in-oil emulsions are made of water drops scattered within an oily base.

EMULSIONS

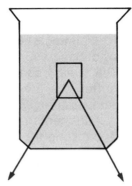

Types	OIL-IN-WATER (O/W)	WATER-IN-OIL (W/O)

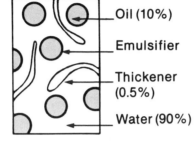

Oil (10%)
Emulsifier
Thickener (0.5%)
Water (90%)

Water (10%)
Emulsifier
Oil (90%)

Important Features	"Break" on contact to release the following:	Help to prevent moisture loss from the skin.
	1. Moisture to enter skin. (softtens, helps overcome dryness.)	Useful for removing grime from skin.
	2. Oils remain on skin surface. (Reduces loss of moisture, lubricates skin.	Cannot be diluted by added water. *(Test for W/O emulsions.)*
	Can be easily diluted by water.	
Examples	Moisturizing Lotion	Cleansing Creams
	Cleansing Lotion	Cold Creams
	Sun Tan Lotion	Night Creams
	Vanishing Cream	Massage Creams

Note: The percentage of water and oil in a product will vary, depending on the formulation of the product and the texture (such as cream or liquid) that is desired.

CAUTION: *Patients should wait 24 hours before applying these products.*

Ointments. Ointments *(OINT ments)* are semisolid mixtures of organic substances (petrolatum or wax) and **medicinal** *(meh DIS i nahl)* agents. No water is present. For the ointment to soften, its melting point should be below that of the body temperature (98.6° F; 37° C).

Ointments are prepared by melting the organic substances and mixing the medicinal agent into the mixture.

Pastes. Pastes are soft, moist cosmetics, having a thick consistency. They are bound together with the aid of gum, starch and water. If oils and fats are present, water is absent.

Examples of Pharmaceutical Preparations

Alcohol, also known as grain or **ethyl** *(ETH il)* alcohol, is a colorless liquid obtained by the **fermentation** *(fur men TAY shun)* of certain sugars. It is a powerful antiseptic and **disinfectant** *(dis in FEK tant).* A 70% solution is most commonly used in electrology for **sanitizing** *(SAN i teyez ing)* instruments, and a 60% solution can be applied to the skin. It is also widely used in perfumes, lotions and tonics.

Ammonia water, as commercially used, is a colorless liquid with a **pungent** *(PUN jent),* penetrating odor. It is a by-product of the manufacture of coal gas. Because it readily dissolves grease, it is used as a cleansing agent. A 28% solution of ammonia gas dissolved in water is available commercially.

Sodium carbonate (washing soda) is prepared by heating **sodium bicarbonate** *(SOH dee um beye KAHR bo nayt).* It is used to soften water, and may also be used with boiling water in the sterilization of metallic instruments. A small quantity is added to the water to keep the instruments bright.

Boric acid, also called boracic acid, is a powder obtained from **sodium borate** *(SOH dee um BOHR art),* which is mined in the form of borax **crystallized** *(KRIS tahl eyezd)* with sulfuric acid. It a mild healing and antiseptic agent. It is sometimes used as a dusting powder, and, in solution, as a cleansing lotion or eyewash.

Glycerine is a sweet, colorless, odorless, syrupy liquid, formed by the **decomposition** *(dee kom po ZISH un)* of oils, fats or molasses. It is a skin softener, and is an ingredient of facial creams and lotions.

Zinc oxide is a heavy white powder made by burning zinc carbonate with coal in a special furnace. It is used as a dusting powder and as an ointment for some skin conditions.

DEPILATORIES

Depilatories *(de PIL ah tohr ees)* are preparations used for the temporary removal of superfluous hair. They consist of various alkali sulfides, **calcium thioglycolate** *(KAL si um theye oh GLEYE coh layt)* compounds, or resins and waxes. They are available in liquid, soft cream, honey, cream, paste, powder or hard cake form.

Before application, a small patch test is done on the patient's skin with the depilatory. If skin redness or blisters **do not** develop, it is safe to use the depilatory over a larger skin surface.

Chemical Type

The **chemical type** of depilatory has the odor of spoiled eggs and is generally used over the legs and arms. It softens and dissolves the hair at the surface of the skin. To prevent irritation of the skin, use only as directed by the manufacturer.

Wax Type

The **heated wax type** of depilatory is odorless and is preferred for the face, legs and bikini line. After the melted wax with an embedded cloth hardens on the hairy surface, the patch is suddenly removed and with it, the hairs. Be sure to follow manufacturer's directions. Cold wax depilatories are also available.

PREPARATIONS FOR SKIN AND FACE

Grouped under this heading are all preparations designed to render the skin or face more attractive in appearance, or to make the patient more comfortable before or after treatment by soothing his or her skin. For these purposes creams, lotions, powders, makeup cosmetics and other products are available.

Creams

Of all preparations used on the skin or face, **creams** are the largest and most varied group. Basically, creams are either stable emulsions of oily and watery substances, or are ointment bases without water.

KIND	COMMON INGREDIENTS	USES
Cold cream	Beeswax, vegetable or mineral oil, water and perfurme	Suitable for cleansing dry or normal skin.
Liquefying cleansing cream	Mineral oil, petrolatum, mineral wax, perfume, small amount of water.	May be used on oily skin. Melts quickly, does not penetrate the skin.
Emollient cream	Waxes, lanolin, vegetable fats and oils, fatty acids, alcohols, and some mineral oil products.	Slightly penetrates and softens the skin. Used for the lubrication of the skin.
Moisturizer	Emollient cream base containing moisturizing agents, PEGs, oils and humectants.	For dryness in aging skin due to lack of moisture and natural oil.

Lotions   **Lotions** are popular products used to a considerable extent in various kinds of treatment. They are available as clear solutions or as suspensions, which have an insoluble sediment at the bottom of the container.

KIND	COMMON INGREDIENTS	USES
Cleansing Lotions	Alcohol or a sulfonated compound, surfactants.	For oily skin
Astringent lotions	Alcohols, witch hazel, in solution of water and glycerine.	For oily skin and large pores.
Skin freshener lotions	Witch hazel, alcohol, mild organic acids, perfume and coloring	Slightly astringent solution for dry skin.
Witch hazel	A solution of alcohol and water containing the astringent from witch hazel	Used as an astringent and cooling lotion.
Calamine lotion	Suspension of prepared calamine and zinc oxide in glycerin, bentonite and lime water.	Used as a soothing application to irritated surfaces of the skin as a protective lotion.
Medicated lotions	Antiseptics, sulfur compounds, or other medicinal agents.	Recommended by a physician for acne or other skin eruptions.

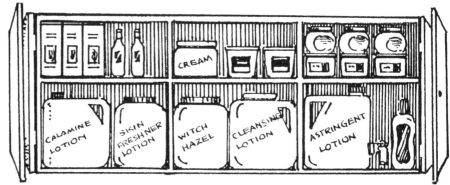

LAWS GOVERNING MANUFACTURE OF PREPARATIONS

There is a tremendous variety of treatment preparations available today. Sales of these products have soared into billions of dollars per year. Because of the growing use of cosmetic preparations, there has been an increase in efforts to protect the consumer from harmful and impure ingredients. In 1938 the Food, Drug and Cosmetic Act was passed by Congress. This act made the manufacturer responsible for product safety and correct labeling. The Fair Packaging and Labeling Act was enacted by Congress in 1966. This act required the identification of the product by name, place of manufacture, net quantity of the contents of the container, and other pertinent information. Such rules and regulations protect the consumer, who may be allergic to certain ingredients, and provide information that is of interest to the electrologist.

The Food and Drug Administration (FDA) is the federal regulatory agency that is responsible for enforcing rules and regulations regarding products (foods, drugs, cosmetics) for public consumption, and is a division of the U.S. Department of Health, Education and Welfare.

The FDA can take legal action against a manufacturer if its product can be proven to be dangerous. The FDA does not take the responsibility of reviewing or testing products before they are distributed to the public, however. Manufacturers must take responsibility for the quality and safety of their products and the claims which they make about those products.

COSMETIC LABELING

To become more familiar with the contents of various preparations now available, the electrologist should carefully read the labels on all products and study their claims.

As of January 1976, the FDA has required that ingredients contained in cosmetic preparations be listed on the labels. Any ingredient that is considered a drug must be listed ahead of the other ingredients. It is essential to read labels and to follow directions for the use of all preparations. This will help you to protect patients from adverse reactions to products and will prevent the misuse of products. For example, the eyes and areas around the eyes are very sensitive, even a mild astringent may cause irritation if allowed to seep into the eyes.

REACTIONS TO PREPARATIONS

There are different kinds of reactions to cosmetics. Some products may cause an irritation, others may cause an allergic reaction. An irritation is easier to deal with than an allergic reaction, which may require extensive testing to find the substance that is causing the reaction. Fragrances and **preservatives** *(pree ZUR vah tivs)* are among the most common allergens.

Many patients will have a **superficial** *(soo per FISH al)* infection if they apply makeup to an area that has just been treated. Reactions to preparations may be detected immediately after application, or the reaction may occur several days later. Symptoms of irritation or allergic reaction are inflammation of the skin, a burning or itching sensation, blisters, blotches, or a rash.

When an irritating or allergy-causing substance has been used near the eyes, they may become swollen, puffy, and tearing may occur.

All preparations and cosmetic products should be kept out of the reach of children.

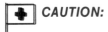 **CAUTION:** *If a patient is allergic to some ingredients in a product and has an adverse reaction that requires medical treatment, the manufacturer of the product is responsible, and is insured to cover possible claims. If the product is formulated in the electrology office, the office will be responsible. Malpractice insurance does not cover medicated or cosmetic products formulated in the office. Therefore it is not a good policy to make and package cosmetics for resale in the office.*

The electrologist may want to familiarize him or herself with the United States Pharmacopeia (U.S.P.), a book defining and standardizing drugs.

QUESTIONS FOR REVIEW

1. What is chemistry?
2. What are elements, compounds and mixtures?
3. What is the difference between physical and chemical change?
4. What is one of the chief characteristics of oxygen?
5. How is pH of a product important?
6. Why is water necessary in electrology reactions?
7. What is a solution?
8. What are the active ingredients of depilatories?
9. What did the Food, Drug and Cosmetic Act of 1938 do?
10. Why is it essential for the electrologist to read labels and follow directions for the use of all preparations?
11. What are the most common allergens in cosmetic preparations?

Chapter 4 Electrology Equipment and Accessories

LEARNING OBJECTIVES   Successful mastery of the material in this chapter will be indicated when you can:

1. List the equipment and accessories necessary for a well-run electrology office.
2. Name the current that electrolysis epilators use.
3. Explain the basic controls on a thermolysis epilator.
4. Name the process which utilizes dual epilators.
5. Describe the proper needle tip.
6. List accessories that will provide patient comfort during electrology treatment.
7. List two uses for small scissors during electrology treatments.
8. Explain the importance of the magnifying mirror.

INTRODUCTION   Sophisticated equipment can never replace your knowledge and skill as an electrologist. It is important that you understand the equipment you choose to use; you must know its capacities and its limitations.

TREATMENT ESSENTIALS   You will need the following equipment and accessories to establish an electrology practice:

1. Galvanic, or shortwave, or dual epilators
2. Needles
3. Patient chair and/or table
4. Electrologist's stool
5. Antiseptic solution
6. Sterilizer
7. Sterile cotton
8. Facial tissue
9. Protective eye-shields for patients sensitive to light
10. Magnification mirror or regular mirror
11. Magnification treatment lamp or glasses
12. Tweezers
13. Apron to cover patient
14. Aftertreatment lotion
15. Small blunt-end scissors
16. Small treatment pillow
17. Covered waste container

NOTE: *A proficient office should have at least double of all the most necessary accessories and equipment in case of unexpected breakdowns or need; especially lamps, epilators, needle holders, needles and foot pedals.*

ELECTROLYSIS EPILATORS   Electrolysis epilators use **galvanic** *(gal VAN ik)* or direct current. The electrical energy may be from a battery or may be converted from alternating current.

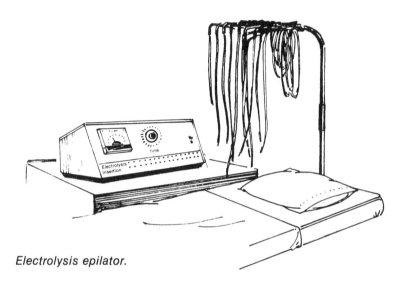

Electrolysis epilator.

Galvanic Controls   All galvanic equipment has the same basic controls. They are:

1. Plug to power source.
2. On/Off switch.
3. **Milliamperemeter** *(MIL i am PEER mee tur)*—gauge which measures galvanic current.
4. **Rheostat** *(REE o stat)*—resistor which controls galvanic current flow.
5. **Positive jack**—electrode that is either attached to or held by the patient.
6. **Negative jack**—receptacle that contains the needle holders.
7. **Indicator light**—shows whether the machine is on or off.
8. **Foot pedal**—starts the current flow when depressed.
9. **Cataphoresis roller** *(KAT oh fo REE sis)*—attachment to the positive jack.

   The galvanic **modality** *(moh DAHL i tee)* of permanent hair removal is used by a very small percentage of electrologists practicing today. Although manufacturers have recently developed more sophisticated galvanic equipment such as computerized epilators, the use of the galvanic method has not substantially increased.

THERMOLYSIS EPILATORS

Thermolysis epilators *(thur MOL i sis EH pil ay tors)* are also known as shortwave epilators. They use radio frequency and operate on alternating current.

Thermolysis is today's most utilized modality for permanent hair removal. Thermolysis became very popular in the late 1940s and has all but replaced the galvanic method since then.

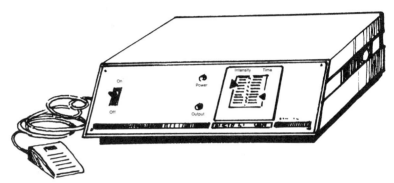

Thermolysis epilator.

Thermolysis Controls

Thermolysis epilators have the same basic controls as galvanic epilators. They are:

1. Plug to power source.
2. On/Off switch.
3. Timer or manual switch.
4. **Intensity control**—regulates current flow (rheostat).
5. **Needle holder jack** (negative electrode).
6. **Foot pedal**—on/off current flow.
7. **Indicator light.**
8. **Intensity light**—indicates pedal is depressed.
9. **Timer light.**

Epilators display the words "FCC (Federal Communications Commission) approved." This does not refer to approval of the effectiveness of the machine. The FCC allows only three frequencies for electrology epilators—13.56, 27.12 and 40.08 megahertz—to be used.

Beyond the basic controls, each manufacturer may add their own innovations. Some, for example, have incorporated two negative jacks to allow needle holders for different sized needles. Other models have RF (Radio Frequency) meters.

Each manufacturer includes an instruction manual with their epilator. Always follow the manufacturer's instructions for use, and your instructor's directions for electrology procedures.

DUAL EPILATORS

The combination of the two currents, direct and alternating, was developed by Henri E. St. Pierre and Arthur Hinkel in 1948. The process became known as the blend.

Dual epilators combine the controls of both the galvanic and thermolysis modalities, and usually include two foot pedals. Some manufacturers have developed a "sequential process" for dual epilators. Again, be guided by the manufacturer or your instructor.

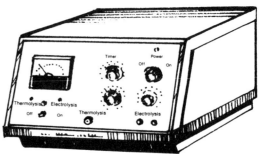

Dual epilator

NEEDLES
It is important to remember that the needle is inserted into the negative needle holder cord electrode. The needle conducts the electricity which causes the action needed in all modalities of treatment. Gold and platinum would be the best conductors, but for economic reasons, surgical stainless steel is used. Insulated needles cannot be used for galvanic or blend methods of electrology. The insulation deteriorates.

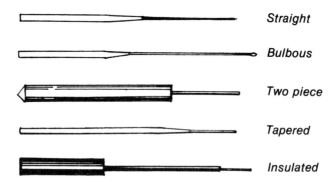

Straight

Bulbous

Two piece

Tapered

Insulated

Needle Tips
The tip of a needle should never be sharply pointed. Such needles could rupture the follicle wall easily, which would make the treatment ineffective and painful, and could cause inflammation.

A needle whose tip is too blunt could also cause problems and make insertions difficult.

The proper tip is ground smooth, and is rounded. It is easiest to analyze the needle tip under 10X magnification.

Needle Diameter
The diameter of the needle used in treatment depends upon the diameter of the hair. Manufacturers produce needle sizes from .001" to .007", .001" being the smallest available. The .001" and .007" are very rarely, if ever, used in treatments today. the .001" and .002" are too narrow in diameter for most treatment, and are prone to breakage. The .007", on the other hand, is too large for most follicles.

The diameter of the needle is equal from the tip to the shank, except in the case of the tapered needle, which is larger at the shank and smaller at the tip.

Needle Sanitation

The most common antiseptic used by electrologists is 70% isopropyl alcohol. In Chapter 9 we will discuss antiseptics and sterilization in detail. It is important to know that these solutions must be used to prepare the needles and the patient before treatment. Antiseptic solutions should be applied only with sterile cotton.

PATIENT COMFORT DURING TREATMENT

The care and comfort of the patient should always be of utmost importance to the electrologist. The comfort of the electrologist is also important. The treatment given will be better quality if the electrologist is comfortable.

Patient Chair or Table

The type of patient chair or table used is determined by the preference of the electrologist, the area of the body to be treated, and the comfort of the patient. Many manufacturers and suppliers now offer a patient chair that folds out into a table.

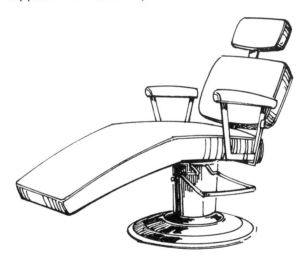

Small Pillow

The pillow is strictly for the patient's comfort. It may be used behind the head or neck, under the arm during treatment, and sometimes under the leg or legs.

Apron To Cover Patient

The apron is used to protect the patient's clothes and to collect the epilated hairs.

After Treatment Lotions

A good antibiotic or antiseptic solution will soothe the area treated, help prevent infection, and aid the healing process. Some are tinted with flesh tones to cover the treated area as well.

Electrologist's Stool

Good work cannot be accomplished if the practitioner is uncomfortable. It is recommended that the electrologist use a chair that has a back rest and that can be easily raised and lowered.

TWEEZERS AND SMALL SCISSORS

Tweezers will be necessary to remove epilated hairs. Small scissors will often be used to cut hair prior to treatment.

Tweezers

There are a variety of tweezers available. The one chosen is a matter of the electrologist's preference and technique. A blunt end tweezer should be used to clean and straighten needles.

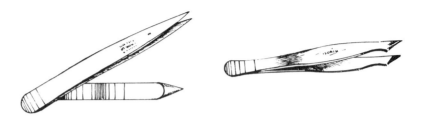

Small Scissors

Small scissors with blunt ends are used to cut extra long eyebrows. Cutting is also necessary when treating areas of the body with long hair such as hairlines, inner thighs, legs, arms and underarms. This will allow the area to be clearly seen so that the angle of growth can be properly judged for good insertions.

MAGNIFICATION MIRRORS, LAMPS AND GLASSES

Magnification equipment will make the electrologist's job much easier and will improve treatment accuracy.

Magnification Mirror

A mirror is essential. Patients will use the mirror to point out the exact area to be treated. The patient can use the mirror to check the area of treatment. When reshaping the hairline and eyebrows, for example, it is a good idea to have the patient use a mirror to watch progress.

Magnification Lamp

A magnification treatment lamp has a magnification glass attached to it which the electrologist looks through to visually enlarge the area to be treated.

Magnification Glasses

Some electrologists wear magnification glasses, used in conjunction with a separate lamp instead of utilizing a magnification lamp.

QUESTIONS FOR REVIEW

1. What equipment and accessories are necessary to the well-run electrology practice?
2. What current does an electrolysis epilator use?
3. What are the basic controls on a thermolysis epilator?
4. What is the name of the process which utilizes dual epilators?
5. What does the proper needle tip look like?
6. What accessories and equipment help provide patient comfort?
7. What are two uses of small scissors during electrology treatments?
8. Why is a magnifying mirror essential?

Chapter 5 Techniques and Procedures

LEARNING OBJECTIVES

Successful mastery of the material in this chapter will be indicated when you can:

1. Explain two key factors for successful epilation.
2. Perform classroom experiments for validating key epilation factors.
3. List the procedures for all three modalities of epilation.
4. Explain factors determining the intensity and time necessary for epilation.
5. List treatment area factors for all areas of the body treated.

INTRODUCTION

Patient safety and quality of treatment are of primary concern to the electrologist. The selection of the proper needle, the intensity and timing of current, and *the exact angle and depth of insertion* are the vital areas of expertise that the student must acquire. These requirements, combined with sensitive touch, finger and hand control, tweezer manipulation, and correct positioning of the patient are the necessary elements for proper treatment.

The most critical procedure in electrology is **proper insertion.** It is therefore wise to practice insertions many hours per day during your electrology course.

EPILATION FACTORS
Point Effect

High-frequency current tends to accumulate at the furthest tip of a conductor—in this case, the tip of the needle. Current also tends to be most intense at the narrowest point of the conductor, or needle.

Moisture Variance

In electrology the extent of tissue destruction is directly related to the amount of moisture present. The skin becomes less moist as it reaches the surface. Therefore, shallow hair follicles contain less moisture than the terminal hair follicles, which are located deeper in the skin.

EXPERIMENTS   In order to examine the point effect of thermolysis and the moisture variance, conduct the following experiments:

Place an egg white in a small glass container. Place a strip of aluminum foil over the edge of the container, touching the egg white and the aluminum foil covering table (see illustration.) Grasp the container at the foil to create an electrical ground. Turn the thermolysis epilator on and place the timer and intensity at very low settings.

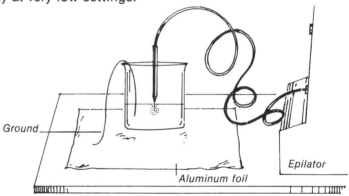

Ground

Aluminum foil

Epilator

Now, test the **coagulation** *(koh ag yoo LAY shun)* patterns the needle makes as the current is activated. Use different needle shapes, time durations, and intensities. A piece of moist meat may also be used to examine the coagulation effects produced by the radio frequency (r.f.) field.

Straight Needle

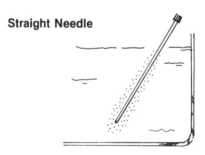

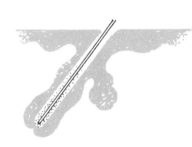

Moisture in hair follicle concentrates energy as shown.

Note the even coagulation of the egg.

Tapered Needle

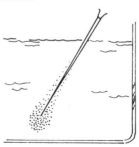

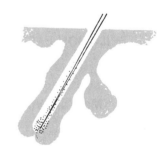

The egg is coagulated at the needle tip.

Concentration is even greater in the follicle.

Bulbous Needle

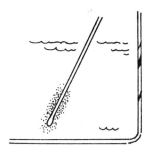 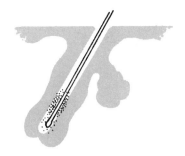

*The egg coagulates above
the bulb.*

*Most of the energy is above the
papilla.*

Insulated Needle

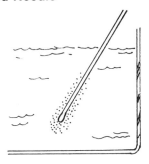 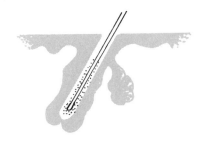

*The egg is coagulated at
the tip.*

*Concentration of energy is
even greater at the tip.*

NOTE: *In order to obtain the "point effect" at the tip of any needle, the intensity must be sufficient to push the energy field to the tip of the needle.*

A **straight needle** does the job very well. A patient who is not very sensitive will not notice the difference between one needle and another. It is always wise to develop a technique that seeks comfort, safety, and effectiveness.

The **tapered needle,** has all the qualities necessary to ensure the point effect. It can produce the required effects at the lower portion of the hair follicle without the use of the high-intensity current required by the insulated probe.

The **bulbous *(BOL bus)* needle** has gone in and out of vogue over the years. Its coagulation pattern is similar to that of the straight needle. According to manufacturers, the bulb was designed to avoid puncture of the hair follicle and straighten any distorted follicle as it was inserted. Tests show that the bulbous probe reacts the same as a straight needle, because the bulb is too small to make a significant difference.

The **insulated needle** causes less upper follicle tissue destruction. The logical and practical results are less sensation to the patient and little or no aftereffects. After the insulated needle was used for several years, however, the following facts also came to light:

- The insulation tends to wear off the needle after a few hours of use.
- The needle has the tendency to stick to the treated tissue. Constant cleaning of the needle slows down the treatment procedure, and if the practitioner is not careful, the insulation can be peeled off during cleaning.
- Autoclave sterilization tends to remove the insulation.
- In order to get the desired coagulation, the epilator has to be raised to higher intensities, as compared with un-insulated needles. The more concentrated energy causes moisture to heat up so fast that a "snapping" sound is heard as the moisture changes into vapor. This sound is known as **decrepitation** *(dee KREP i TAY shun)*.
- If the intensity is kept low, the lower portion of the hair follicle does not receive as much destruction as the upper portion. This is especially true of the deeper, terminal hair follicles.
- The fine **vellus** *(VEL us)* hair and even fine dark hair with shallow roots is, therefore, not protected by the insulated portion of the needle.
- Experts believe that not only must the dermal papilla be destroyed, but that at least the lower two-thirds of the hair follicle must also be destroyed in order to obtain permanent hair removal. Since the insulated probe concentrates its energy only at the lower quarter of the hair follicle, these experts assume there will be greater regrowth.
- insulation may disintegrate when the needle is used with galvanic current.

  Remember that it is not only the needle that makes the difference; the expertise of the practitioner is even more important.

Diameter of Needle   The diameter of the needle relates directly to the diameter of the hair to be treated. It is commonly taught that the needle size should equal the size of the hair. However, it must be remembered that the thinner the needle, the hotter and more intense the sensation to the patient. The larger the needle diameter, the less pain there will be.

To understand this principle, consider lying on the beach in the warm sun on an 80° day. It is very enjoyable, but if a special scope concentrated all the sun's rays onto one small area of your body, it would burn a severe hole. The sun did not change, but the sun's area of concentration did. This is what happens when an electrologist switches from a large needle to a fine needle without lowering the intensity control.

For this reason, it is wise to select a needle at least one size (.001) larger in diameter than the hair being treated. This will allow for greater comfort to the patient and will permit greater distribution of energy around the dermal papilla, providing the insertion can be made easily. The hair follicle has elasticity and should permit greater diameter needles to enter without force.

Needle Length   The length of the needle will depend on the average depth of the hair follicles in the area to be treated. In general, dark terminal hairs lie deeper than the fine dark and vellus hairs.

To analyze follicle depth, grasp the hair with the tweezer at the surface of the skin and remove it. The distance from the tweezer to the root is the depth of the hair follicle. Select a needle that is slightly longer than the measure depth.

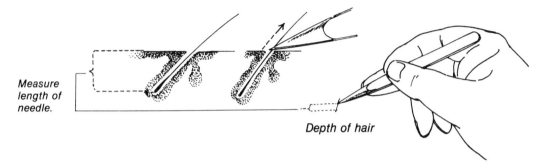

Measure length of needle.

Depth of hair

Today, most needles manufactured are the push-in type, which can be adjusted in and out of the needleholder to a desired length. The screw-on type cannot be adjusted, and therefore, must be chosen according to the manufactured lengths.

After a few years experience, a proficient electrologist will be able to determine the width and length of a needle simply by examining the area to be treated.

 NOTE: *Be sure that current is off during practice procedures.*

The Insertion   The insertion is the most critical technique in electrology treatment. Hold the needleholder as you would a pen or pencil, *but not as firmly.* The index finger and thumb must not touch. The needle holder may lean gently on the middle finger, which serves as a guide.

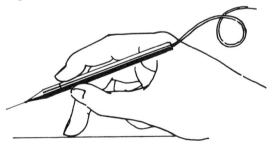

The angle at which the needle is inserted depends on the angle at which the hair is growing. For example, a hair that grows straight up requires the needle to be inserted straight. If a hair is growing at a severe angle, the needle will be inserted at that same angle. If there is an excessive amount of hair and the hair is long, it will be difficult to see the hair follicle and the angle of growth. Simply cut the hair to a length where the follicle and angle of growth can be observed.

NOTE: *Be careful not to touch the needle to the surface of the skin when treating hairs that grow at an angle close to the skin. This can result in unnecessary pain and scabbing.*

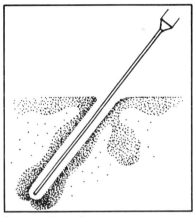

Correct insertion.

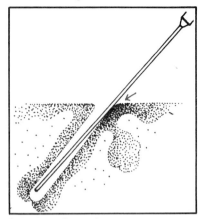

Incorrect insertion.

When you make insertions, keep your arms below shoulder level. If your arms are raised above your shoulders, the blood will rush from them, making them tire quickly. Your insertions will then be much less accurate.

Use a magnifying lamp in order to better see fine, colorless hairs.

When observing the area to be treated, move the lamp into the working area so that one side of the hair is illuminated and the other side is shadowed. Follow your instructor's directions for this technique.

Sometimes a sterile, flesh-colored powder can be used to accentuate the pore. Insert the needle following the angle of hair growth. Gently insert the needle, and if there is any resistance, change your angle of insertion until the needle easily slides into the hair follicle.

On some areas of the body insertions can become quite awkward. For instance, on the neck right below the chin, and in the inner-thigh area. If the hair grows at an angle close to the skin and away from you, a proper insertion becomes difficult, requiring a backhand technique.

Backhand technique

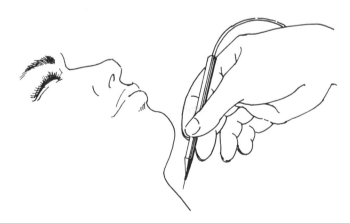

In a case like this, your instructor may suggest you bend the needle to the angle at which the hair is growing. This will avoid unnecessary fatigue. Some manufacturers have introduced a new needle holder that the practitioner can bend easily for difficult-to-reach areas.

The fingers of the free hand are used to position the hair and act as a guide for single or multiple insertions. (Multiple insertions treat several hairs, then remove them with tweezers.) Continue to maintain the fingers of the free hand in the area being treated by multiple insertions. The fingers then become a point of reference for the hairs that have been treated.

The gentle pressure of the fingertips of the free hand properly placed can also alleviate the sensation of the treatment.

Tweezer Manipulation

Once the insertion technique is well developed, the maneuvering of the needleholder and tweezer must be mastered.

The tweezer is held inside the clasped hand with the needleholder. The tweezer is held by the fourth and fifth fingers as the point end extends out between the thumb and first finger.

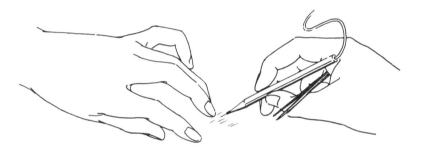

The needleholder and tweezer should not be held tightly. The student must practice a light touch. The patient quickly recognizes a heavy hand.

Time must be taken to practice maneuvering the needleholder and tweezer. The first finger and thumb must exchange the needleholder for the tweezer. The needleholder will slide between fingers two and three and the pointed end of the tweezer will be held lightly by the tips of the thumb and index finger. Now grasp the hair as if to be removed.

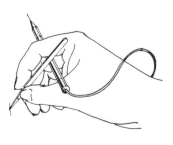

After some proficiency has been developed, we can proceed to practice *with the current on.*

EPILATION PROCEDURES
Thermolysis

Thermolysis (short wave) Procedure:
(Your instructor's procedure is equally correct.)

1. Position aproned patient on chair.
2. Wash your hands.
3. Sanitize area to be treated.
4. Sterilize tweezers.
5. Determine size of needle required and sterilize.
6. Turn epilator on and wait one minute.
7. Set timer on Low.
8. Set intensity on Low.
9. Make first insertion until resistance occurs. Raise the needle very slightly.
10. Depress foot switch.
11. Test hair with tweezer for an easy release.
12. Raise intensity and timer accordingly, until hair is easily released.

INTENSITY-TIME RATIO

The amount of intensity and time necessary is related to the type of hair being treated and the amount of hair to be removed.

The calibrations on the intensity and timer dials are arbitrary measurements for all epilators. They are simply reference points for you to remember when treating similar types of hair with the same epilator. These settings can vary with the moisture content of the patient's skin and the electrical power coming into the epilator at the time of treatment. If the needle-holder cord is lying on the patient's body it could be losing energy, and would also thereby cause the settings to vary. (The setting number can vary from manufacturer to manufacturer.)

Bulb Test

A good technique for determining intensity involves a small 6-watt bulb. Simply hold the screw portion of the bulb with one hand and place the needle on the contact point at the end of the bulb with the other hand. Depress the foot pedal. The bulb will light up. The higher the intensity, the brighter the bulb.

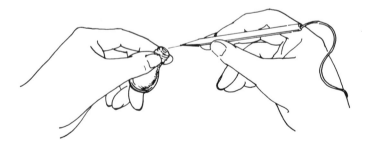

There is no danger in performing this test. You won't feel a thing. After some experience, you will make a mental note of the relationship between the glow and the type of hair to be treated. This technique is also good for determining malfunctions.

CAUTION: Sometimes current is not entering the hair follicle. The tendency is to raise the current. **Do not do this, because it could overtreat the hair follicle.** Use the bulb test to determine if current is flowing. There could be a break in the cord. This usually occurs where the cord enters the needleholder.

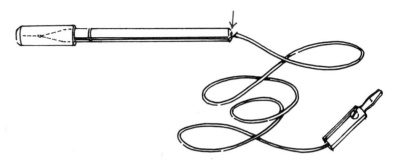

Replace the needleholder cord with a new one immediately, and repeat the bulb test. If the bulb does not lightup, make sure the epilator is plugged in and change the foot pedal. If none of these tests prove positive, the epilator needs service.

The intensity and time ratios can vary from one expert to another. Each school and instructor may have their own theories. Technically speaking, these theories have been reduced to two schools of thought. One is the *instant method,* also known as the *flash method,* and the other is the *slow method,* also known as the *manual method.*

When a patient is receiving treatment he or she has five main concerns: pain, effectiveness, time, scarring, and cost.

The *instant method* is the one most commonly used. It simply involves *the use of a high intensity combined with a very low time duration.* The time can be as low as one-tenth of a second to one second, enabling the practitioner to treat more hairs in less time. The patient does not have to endure a lengthy sensation per hair. *The time control must be in the On position for the instant method.* Since a high intensity is used in this process, the electrologist must employ the use of the timer to protect against *overtreatment.* The timer automatically shuts off the current.

During treatment the practitioner must note the comfort of the patient, the skin sensitivity, and the type of hair being treated. Lowering the intensity may make the patient more comfortable but the hair may not come out as easily. The point at which the hair will slip out easily while providing maximum comfort to the patient is called **effective treatment setting.**

If the hair is very dense, spread the treatment out. Do not treat hairs that are close to each other. Following this procedure will prevent the skin from becoming too inflamed, and will allow it to heal more rapidly.

After 10 to 15 minutes of treatment, most patients will witness a numbness in the area being treated. This phenomenon will be discussed later when the physiology *(fiz i OL o jee)* and histology *(hi STOL o jee)* of the skin and hair are described.

During the treatment, redness will occur. This is normal. It is a result of the blood rushing to the treated area and is not cause for alarm. A snapping sound indicates that the moisture reached the gaseous state instantaneously. The surface of the skin should not be affected.

 CAUTION: *When using the* **instant method,** *remember to lower the intensity as the hairs become finer and the follicles more shallow. As the hairs become thicker and the follicles deeper, the hairs will not slip out after treatment. The electrologist then will increase the intensity until the hair slides out easily.*

Electro-coagulation *(i LEK troh koh AG yoo LAY shun)* The instant method will coagulate the tissue in the lower portion of the hair follicle at 127° to 129° F. (60° to 61°C). This action will destroy the living cells responsible for hair growth.

Electro-desiccation *(i LEK troh DES i KAY shun).* When the intensity reaches 212° F (100°C), or the boiling point, the water quickly evaporates into a gas and will desiccate *(DES i KAYT)* (dehydrate) the tissue surrounding the dermal papilla. This causes more damage to the tissue than electro-coagulation. In order to avoid overtreatment, the timer control must be set very low.

Developing an expert's skill of insertion and correctly using the instant method will decrease the pain and increase the efficiency of the treatment.

Slow Method. The slow method, once known as the manual method, uses a low intensity of current and a longer treatment time. The duration is usually 5 to 20 seconds per hair.

The theory in this procedure is that the high-frequency current action creates more tissue destruction surrounding the entire length of the needle.

Caution must be used with this procedure as the current is manually controlled. Turn the timer switch to Off, or put it in the manual position. Insert the needle and begin to increase intensity until the patient feels a sensation. After 5 to 10 seconds, try to remove the hair. If it does not slip out easily, try another 5 seconds. Once the hair slides out easily, remove it and go on to the next. If the hair does not come out easily, tweeze it and go on to the next hair to avoid overtreatment.

In both the slow method and the instant method, the standard of epilation is the removal of the treated hair without forced tweezing.

Electrolysis
(Galvanism)
As we have discussed, the galvanic method has been almost completely replaced by the thermolysis method. In recent years, however, manufacturers have introduced innovative, computerized galvanic epilators and epilators with dual modalities. It is, therefore, appropriate to understand the procedures for galvanic treatment.

Electrolysis (galvanism) Procedure:

1. Position aproned patient on chair or table.
2. Patient must be in good contact with positive electrode.
3. Wash your hands.
4. Select the appropriate size needles and insert them into the amount of needleholders you intend to use, depending on the particular epilator and individual procedure.
5. Sterilize the needles and disinfect the area to be treated.
6. Turn the epilator on and wait 1 minute.
7. Insert the first needle.
8. Step on foot pedal and watch the milliamperemeter *(mil ee AM per mee ter)* until it reads 3/10 of a milliampere.
9. Test hair after 60 seconds for easy removal. Continue to test for up to 2 minutes until hair slips out easily.
10. Try to increase the intensity to a point where the patient can easily tolerate the sensation. This will enable you to reduce the amount of time necessary to epilate the hair properly.

Some new epilators will time the hairs individually and shut off automatically, making overtreatment impossible. Various manufacturers have different operating procedures. Check with the owner's manual or your instructor for details.

Electrolysis treatment causes a chemical destruction of the hair follicle. The sodium hydroxide in solution can last for a short time after the current is off and continue its action.

Dual Method
(Thermolysis and
Electrolysis)

The dual method incorporates the advantages of both thermolysis and electrolysis currents, together or sequentially, with separate foot pedals.

Dual method (thermolysis and electrolysis) Procedure:

Once again, each manufacturer has specific procedures. We will discuss the general technique used. Consult your instructor for additional directions.

1. Position aproned patient on chair or table.
2. Make sure patient is in good contact with positive electrodes.
3. Wash your hands.
4. Select the appropriate size needle.
5. Sterilize needle and sanitize area to be treated.
6. Turn epilator On and wait 1 minute.
7. Insert needle.
8. Using the slow method, depress the thermolysis foot pedal and treat the hair for easy removal, up to 10 seconds on a very low intensity.
9. If hair does not come out easily, tweeze it and go on to the next hair, raising the intensity another unit. You are trying to find the ***effective treatment setting.***
10. Testing again, count to yourself how many seconds it takes to epilate the hair. Do not go over 10 seconds. Once the ***effective treatment setting*** for thermolysis is determined, you can incorporate the galvanic current.

11. Insert the needle into a hair follicle with a hair of similar diameter, but now depress both pedals for 6 to 7 seconds, making sure the milliamperemeter reaches at least 7/10.
12. When hair slips out, stop the thermolysis and continue with the galvanic for at least another 2 seconds.

The time necessary for the galvanic to be effective is reduced substantially because the heat of the thermolysis causes the caustic effect of the sodium hydroxide to increase approximately 15 times.

Manufacturers of blend equipment alternate the currents according to their own theories. Your instructor will be able to help you evaluate the validity of each manufacturer's approach.

Modality Conclusions. It is very evident that slow thermolysis, electrolysis, and dual methods will all cause great tissue destruction. This should permit an increase in effectiveness. *Remember that all modalities and techniques rate their effectiveness by the smooth and easy removal of the hair from the treated follicle.* The electrologist must determine, then, if the time lost during the slow manual method, electrolysis, or the dual method is worth the extra sensitivity for the patient to gain a theoretical increase in effectiveness. Time, cost, and pain are also concerns of the patient. Each must be considered when choosing treatment modality.

TREATMENT AREA FACTORS

Each area of the body will require different procedures, techniques, and positioning. We will start with areas of the head and continue downward.

Hairline

The hairline or forehead can be a problem area for men as well as women. An irregular hairline or one that almost meets the eyebrows is unsightly.

SATT
Suggested Area Treatment Time
Up to 1 hour.

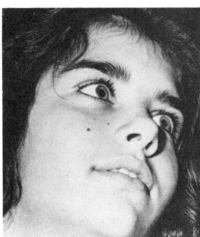 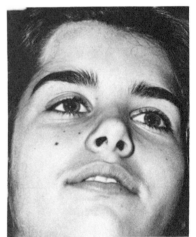

Hair Transplants
SATT
Suggested Area Treatment Time
Up to 1 hour.

Another unique problem in recent years is the treatment of hair plugs. Hair plugs are groupings of hair follicles removed from the nape of a person's neck and surgically reimplanted into the balding area.

Some patients do not like how the transplant looks or feels. The new hairline is not natural looking. So, they seek the electrologist's help in designing a proper line of growth. Treat only the hairs in the front row of plugs on the first treatment.

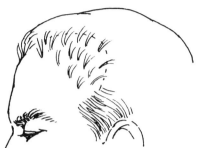

An example of hair transplants.

In all cases of hairline treatment, there must be an agreement on what exactly the patient wants. A talented and artistically minded electrologist will be able to assist the patient in making a decision.

In some cases, the patient may be extremely nervous. He or she may be afraid the treated area will come out looking bad. In a case like this, it may be necessary to cut the hair first and show very clearly what the hairline will look like after the treatment is complete.

To begin treatment on an uneven hairline, simply wet the area thoroughly with an antiseptic solution. Also wet the frontal hairs that will not be treated. If the hairs are long, cut them to a length that will enable you to determine the angle of growth. Cut only the hairs you plan to remove during that particular treatment.

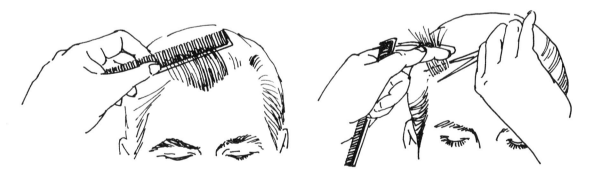

Treating the uneven hairline.

Proceed to remove hairs starting from the front end and moving back row by row. Be careful not to make the hairline too even, otherwise it will look artificial. As you reach the normal hairline, thin the growth. Thin the hairline about a quarter inch into the scalp. Every so often allow the patient to see the progress and offer suggestions.

Completing treatment of a hairline is one of the most gratifying experiences for both the patient and the electrologist. The patient will receive compliments on how good he or she looks, and people will not be able to tell what made the difference.

Eyebrows

SATT

Suggested Area
Treatment Time

Up to 1 hour.

Eyebrows shaping is a service sought by men as well as women. The bridge of the nose, the area between the eyebrows, is the problem in most cases.

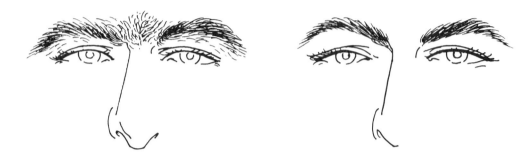

The bridge of the nose is fairly simple to treat. The most important thing to remember is to agree with the patient on exactly where they wish the beginning of their eyebrows to be. This is usually in line with the corner of the eye. Once this point is established, thin the area so it will not become too inflamed. When treating men, it is a good idea to leave some of the finer hairs behind. To make an eyebrow perfectly clear could give a feminine appearance which the male may not want.

When treating the lid or the area beneath the brow, use an eyebrow comb dampened with alcohol and comb upward. This will allow you to see the superfluous hair beneath the eyebrow which must be removed. Once again, thin out the area to avoid overtreatment.

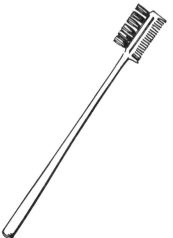

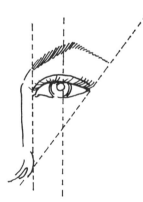

Note the natural line as you comb upward.

Align a pencil along dotted lines to determine ideal brow shape.

The shape of the eyebrow will become self-evident during the combing. A talented electrologist will be able to assist the patient with shaping. It is best to avoid overthinning the eyebrows.

Eyebrow comb

The area above the eyebrow is also important. Comb the eyebrow down. The hairs that do not fall into the eyebrow line will be evident. Remove these hairs, allowing the patient to confirm your decision.

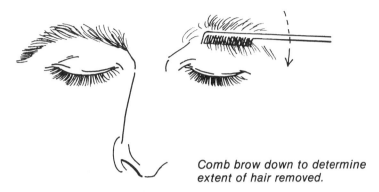

Comb brow down to determine extent of hair removed.

After approximately age 35, both men and women experience a change in the eyebrow-hair growth cycle. Some of the hairs will grow thicker and longer. A few of these hairs may be removed permanently. If there are many, however, it is best to trim them. Otherwise you would make the eyebrow appear too sparse. Do not trim the hairs below the eyebrow line. To do so would make the eyebrow appear unnatural.

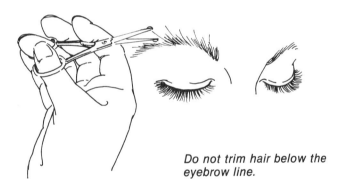

Do not trim hair below the eyebrow line.

It is important to remember that the eyebrows are densely populated with surface capillaries *(KAP i ler ee)*. If an improper insertion is made, a black and blue mark will appear, indicating that a capillary was punctured. Apply ice and inform the patient that the lid will clear within a week or so.

Upper Lip

SATT
Suggested Area
Treatment Time
15 to 20 minutes.

The upper lip is probably the most common area of treatment. The lip is also one of the most sensitive areas to treat. In most cases, it reddens very quickly, and might embarrass the patient in public. There is also a chance that the lip will swell. This is why it is best to limit lip treatments to 15 to 20 minutes. First, thin the hair during treatments to decrease irritation. While the aftereffects are only short-term and cosmetic in nature, your patient will appreciate your efforts to avoid them as much as possible.

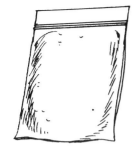

Apply small ice packs to reduce inflammation and soothe patient.

The immediate application of small sanitized ice packs will reduce the inflammation to a minimum. Fill small clear plastic jewelry bags with water and freeze them. Give these frozen packets to those patients who seem to react or who wish to hold something cool on the treated areas as they leave your office.

During treatment, ask your patient to avoid tweezing or bleaching. He or she may cut the hairs if desired. It is important that the patient keep a schedule of treatments, as hair treated in the early stages of growth (anagen) *(AN ah jen)* have shallower follicles and are easier to treat, giving better results.

Top of Nose
SATT
Suggested Area
Treatment Time
5 minutes.

In most cases, the top of the nose grows only a few hairs that usually appear later in life. The hairs are generally dark and fine. They are shallow, but must be treated carefully to avoid pitting and large scabbing.

 CAUTION: *Never treat the inside of the nose.*

Sides of Face
SATT
Suggested Area
Treatment Time
30 minutes per side.

The sides of the face, including the sideburns, can be a time consuming area to treat. The length of treatment will depend on the amount of hair, its texture, the sensitivity of the skin, and the sensitivity of the patient to pain.

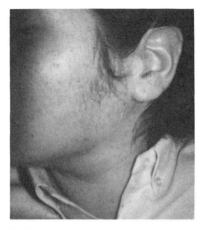
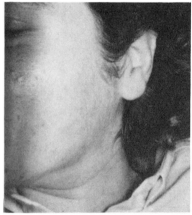

Before   *After*

It is important once again to thin the areas, trying not to treat hairs that are too close together. This will prevent overtreatment, especially on the face, which cannot be readily concealed.

If the hair is too long to treat, cut it. This will allow you to see the angle of growth more easily, and will make the patient feel more presentable.

Remove the darkest and heaviest growth first. The patient will then see immediate progress. It is best to limit the first treatment to 15 minutes on each side of the face. The first treatment will enable you to establish how sensitive the skin is and help you determine the time of succeeding treatments. If the patient is extremely sensitive, your instructor may direct you to remove the fine hairs first, so that the numbing of the area will permit the patient to tolerate treatment of the terminal hairs.

When treating the sideburn, make sure that you and the patient agree where the hairline will end.

Chin

SATT
Suggested Area
Treatment Time

Up to 45 minutes.

The chin is probably the second most common area to be treated. It is one of the areas that is most affected by hormone change, especially on women after the age of 35.

The chin causes the most aggravation to the electrologist. This is because the female patient usually grows more new hair in this area as she grows older. The tendency of the patient is to blame the electrologist, not the increase of new hair growth. Since this hair is so obvious, the patient is most sensitive about it. You must be able to explain the situation clearly so she will have confidence in you and your treatment. ("Regrowth" will be discussed further in the chapter entitled "Regrowth and Statistics.") You must explain to her that most of the hair is *new* and only a few are hairs growing from a previously treated hair follicle.

Be careful not to overtreat the chin area. It tends to grow dark, deep terminal hairs close to each other. Overtreatment can cause hyperpigmentation *(HEYE per PIG men TAY shun)* to occur and possible pitting.

Neck—Front and Back

SATT
Suggested Area
Treatment Time

Up to 1 hour.

Hair growing on the neck can be a nuisance to the man as well as to the woman. Many times the unwanted hair on a woman can extend from the chin, neck, chest, right on down to the naval area and the pubic region.

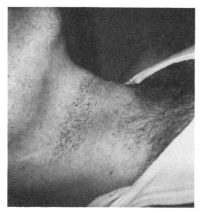
Before

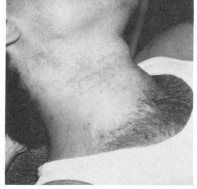
After

Once the neck area is completed, the patient must be advised that it is not unusual to grow more hair in this section as she grows older, usually a few hairs per year, As you begin to treat the neck area and the body, scabbing will become more prevalent.

Neck—Front and Back
continued

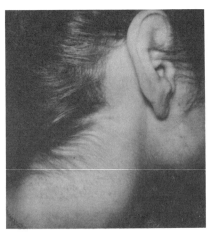

The back of the neck is of concern, especially when the female patient wants a short haircut or wishes to wear her hair up. For the man, this hair is extremely bothersome, especially if there is no division between the back hairline and the hair on the back.

Ears

SATT
Suggested Area
Treatment Time

20 minutes per ear.

The ears can become a problem, especially for older men. The hairs usually grow along the edge of the ear. Some men and women can grow hair as profusely on the ears as they do on the face. The electrologist must be extra patient with the ears. If the insertions are not made properly, they will bleed easily. So take your time and cool the area with antiseptic lotion as you proceed with treatment.

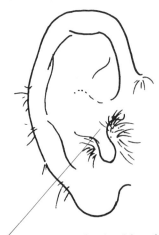

CAUTION: *Do not treat the inside of the ear.*

Breasts

SATT
Suggested Area
Treatment Time

15 minutes.

Most women are frightened to have hairs removed from this area. However, doctors assert that there is no danger, even during pregnancy. In most cases, there are only a few hairs surrounding the nipple or areola area. This is one of the least sensitive areas to treat; however, hairs must be treated very carefully. They must slip out easily, otherwise those that regrow may become ingrown.

Chest

SATT

Suggested Area
Treatment Time

1 hour female;
2 hours male.

Chest hair on women is usually concentrated between the breasts and above. There is no problem removing this growth.

If a man wants treatment in this area, it is best that you ask exactly what he would like accomplished. Usually men want their shoulders and 2 inches (5 cm.) of the chest cleared. Some may want the chest thinned, while others may want all the hair removed. Treat the area proportionately. Never leave a straight line of treatment across the chest. After each treatment, the area should look as natural as possible.

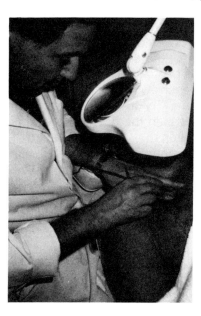 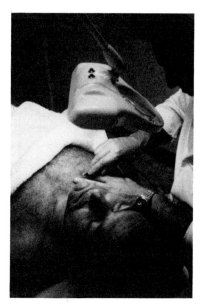

Back

SATT

Suggested Area
Treatment Time

1 to 2 hours female;
1 to 3 hours male.

This area is generally a problem with men. Some women may also develop hair in this area. It is usually concentrated on the small of the lower back above the bathing-suit line.

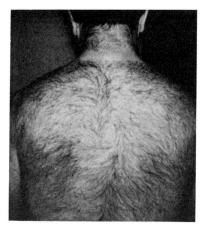 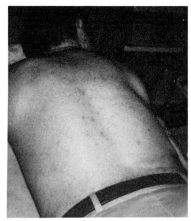

Before   *After*

Arms and Hands

SATT
Suggested Area
Treatment Time
1 hour per arm.

Hair on the arms has been a problem to women for centuries. As electrologists have become better trained and more proficient women have begun to recognize new hope in electrolysis treatment. Years ago, patients thought the arms were too difficult to treat. Today, however, this area can be treated as quickly and safely as any other area of the body.

Before treatment, discuss with the patient the technique you will use. Some will want their hands completed first, while others will want you to thin the arms and hands during each treatment. Whatever technique you use, advise your patient that there will be some scabbing. In some cases, freckles and moles once covered by hair become more evident. Once arms are finished, the skin is clear and permanently smooth.

It is best to thin the arms of the heaviest hairs first and work progressively, using this technique over the entire surface of the arm. Try to work on each arm so one arm does not look clearer than the other. However, some patients prefer that you remain on the same arm instead of change. They may like to see the dramatic difference or feel that to change arms would mean going through the more sensitive portion of treatment all over again.

After arms have been completed, it is important to inform the patient that these areas will now sunburn faster than they did before treatment. The reason is that the hair removed used to filter much of the sun's rays and provided more sebum to cover the skin. After the first season, however, the skin will adjust itself. Suggest that the patient use a good sunscreen to protect these areas before sunbathing.

The electrologist must use extra care when treating these arms as they tend to scab. It's a good idea to space treatments and use a good aftertreatment lotion.

Underarms

SATT
Suggested Area
Treatment Time
30 minutes per underarm.

The underarms can be treated safely. The glands that concern most people lie well beneath the area of treatment.

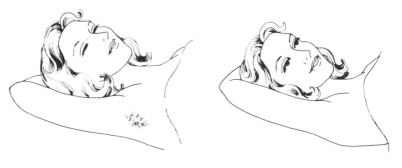

Before   After

Abdomen
SATT
Suggested Area
Treatment Time
45 minutes.

The area above the bathing-suit line is a very common problem. This area tends to grow more hair after puberty, and is very sensitive, tending to scab easily.

Inner Thighs
SATT
Suggested Area
Treatment Time
Up to 1 hour per inner thigh.

The inner thighs or lower bathing-suit line is a very popular area of treatment. Most women have either shaved or waxed this area. Some have found the temporary methods to be bothersome or to cause harsh after-effects, such as ingrown hairs.

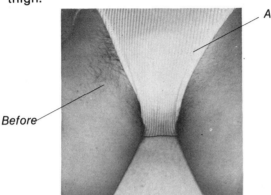

After

Before

This area is sensitive for most women. As treatment progresses, many patients tend to tolerate the sensation better. Work according to the patient's request to determine the amount of time per treatment and time allowed treating each hair. *Once all the hair is removed, it is important to schedule the next appointment within two weeks.* In this way, you will treat hairs in early anagen which will require much less energy to destroy the small dermal papilla. *The treatment will take less time and cause much less sensitivity while assuring greater effectiveness.*

The side-effects of treating this area include: scabbing, possible ingrown hairs, and hyperpigmentation. The patient must be made aware of these temporary cosmetic aftereffects before treatment begins. The effects will disappear and the skin will be smooth and clear of hair forever.

Buttocks
SATT
Suggested Area
Treatment Time
Up to 1 hour.

This area is a concern for both men and women. It can become a problem due to ingrown hair. In fact, many of the pilonidal *(peye toh NEYE dah)* cysts that occur on the lower portion of the spine above the buttocks (or the midline over the saral *(SAH rahl)* area) are nothing more than groups of ingrown hairs. This area can be easily and safely treated without any side effects.

Legs

SATT

Suggested Area
Treatment Time

2 or more hours per leg.

The treatment of legs is becoming more and more popular for men as well as women. Patients should be made aware of the approximate time necessary to complete their legs. Once legs are finished, a periodic cleanup may be necessary every few months for a year or so. Thereafter, the legs will be smooth and permanently hair-free. *Like the arms, the legs will sunburn faster after treatment.*

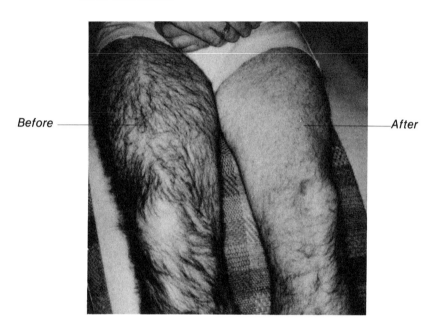

Before ———————————————————————— After

Feet and Toes

SATT

Suggested Area
Treatment Time

15 minutes per foot.

The amount of hair on the feet and toes can vary greatly from person to person. These areas are generally sensitive and tend to scab. Once treated, a few new hairs may grow each year. Eventually, toes and feet will also stay permanently clear.

Eyelashes

If we remember our electrolysis history, eyelash treatment is how the profession came to be. Today, as well as in Dr. Michel's day, the inverted eyelash hair growth is a problem.

Some patients actually have hair growing under the eyelid itself. In others the lids begin to invert due to age, and the lashes begin to irritate the eye. Another problem can occur after plastic surgery, or "eye lifts." The eyelid is sometimes distorted and a few of the lashes are twisted toward the eye.

The process is quite tedious. If your modality is equipped with an air blower, shut it off. Using extra magnification, examine the lid to be treated. Once you've determined the hair to be treated, choose the appropriate needle. Keep your patient calm and relaxed. With your free hand, hold the lid steady and treat the hair or hairs.

Before treatment, it is advisable to check with your insurance company and to learn about the laws for your location.

Special Considerations

Moles. There has been much controversy over whether or not to treat hairy moles. There are no recorded histories of bad side effects due to treatment of a mole. In some cases, it is claimed that the mole has disappeared within months after treatment.

It is suggested that electrologists check with their insurance company and with their state's regulations before treating the hair in moles. Obtain permission from a physician before treating the patient.

Diabetics. A similar controversy exists with treating diabetic patients as with treating moles. The electrologist should consult his or her insurance policy and state regulations before treatment, and should also obtain the physician's permission.

Blacks. There is no problem in treating black patients. Many are concerned with keloids *(KEE loids)* and with distorted hair follicles. Always keep in mind that when a hair regrows in a hair follicle that has been treated previously, it comes in straight and very shallow. This hair can then be treated as you would Caucasian hair.

The after-effects are similar to most treatment, although black skin tends to hyperpigmentate more than white. This does disappear and the skin returns to its original color.

NOTE: *Give a 15 minute test treatment, then check for reaction after one week. If results are satisfactory, proceed with treatment.*

Warts. Do not treat near warts as electrolysis treatment can spread them. Always check with a dermatologist before treating a patient with warts.

Pacemakers. It is possible for electrolysis treatment to interfere with the functioning of a patient's pacemaker. Check the rules and regulations of your state and with your insurance company before treating a patient with a pacemaker. It is also wise to check with the patient's physician.

Some Special Suggestions for Patient Comfort

The following have been found to reduce the sensitivity of patients, and to relax them for treatment.
1. A perfect insertion.
2. The use of ice.
3. Ethyl chloride *(ETH el KLOR eyed)* freeze spray
4. Application of numbing ointments (especially for the lip)
5. Music
6. Television
7. Good conversation (when applicable)
8. Proper finger pressure
9. Treating finer hairs first so that the area becomes numb before proceeding with darker hairs

Aftertreatment Suggestions

1. Caution patient not to let the treated area get sunburned.
2. Caution the patient to avoid using cosmetics for at least 24 hours.
3. Apply only antiseptic solutions or ointments for 24 hours.
4. Use icepacks on sensitive or inflammed areas.
5. Advise patient of all possible after-effects, such as scabbing, swelling, hyperpigmentation, and superficial inflammation. Assure them that all these effects are of a cosmetic nature only.
6. Always show confidence and express how nicely the patient is progressing.
7. Allow enough time for healing before making the next appointment. A week is usually sufficient.

QUESTIONS FOR REVIEW

1. What are the two key factors for successful epilation?
2. What classroom experiments can help you determine how to achieve these key epilation factors?
3. What is the procedure for epilation with thermolysis? For electrolysis? For the dual method?
4. What factors determine the intensity and time necessary for thermolysis?
5. What are treatment area factors to consdider for all areas of the body treated?
6. What glands can cause excess hair?

Chapter 6 Effects of Maltreatment

Successful mastery of the material in this chapter will be indicated when you can:

1. List at least 10 causes of overtreatment.
2. Explain three factors that can result in undertreatment.
3. Discuss three safeguards that can help the electrologist ensure that treatment is adequate.

INTRODUCTION   Professional electrologists, legislators, allied health professionals, and the public all want electrology treatment standards that are clearly defined. They question, "Is it normal to have 20 hours of treatment on the upper lip? Is scarring unavoidable when treating hair which is thick and dark? Will the hair always grow back? What about distorted hair? Can any problem really be solved forever?" Clearly defined guidelines will answer such questions.

All expert electrologists must be able to determine overtreatment, undertreatment, and when an epilator is not effective. It is, therefore, imperative for the student to become aware of all future and past methods, and of all devices that claim to remove hair permanently. (For a detailed discussion on electrolysis equipment, see Chapter 4.)

OVERTREATMENT   Overtreatment is the most severe form of maltreatment. There are several reasons why overtreatment occurs. The main reasons are:

1. Intensity too high in the "instant" or "flash" methods of thermolysis.
2. Timer left on too long or the electrologist did not lift his or her foot from the foot pedal soon enough during the "manual" or "slow" technique.
3. The intensity is either too high and/or the timing is too long when using the blend or dual method.
4. Too shallow an insertion at any intensity with any method.
5. Failure to stop current flow before removing the needle from the hair follicle.
6. The use of a very fine needle without lowering the intensity. This causes pitting.
7. Treating hairs that are too close to each other, which causes inflammation and possible scarring.

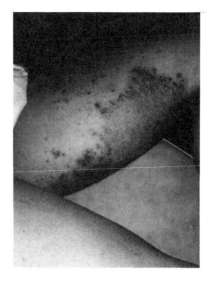
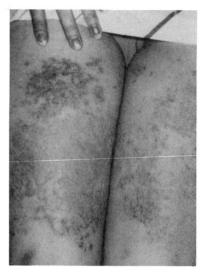
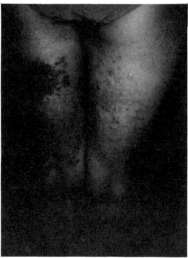

These photos demonstrate very clearly that the electrologist has missed the hair follicle completely. The black and blue marks reveal ruptured capillaries and the severe inflammation discloses the treatment of hairs that were too close to each other. The area is also severely infected, probably due to the lack of sterile procedures.

8. Inserting the needle too deeply, which results in broken follicle walls, ruptured capillaries, and black and blue marks.
9. Missing the hair follicle completely and applying current at the same time. This can cause a permanent pit in the skin and/or black and blue marks.
10. Lack of sanitary procedures.
11. Extra caution must be taken by galvanic and blend practitioners when treating dark, deep terminal hairs. Too much of the lasting sodium hydroxide solution can cause overtreatment.
12. The patient can cause the damage by applying cosmetics and picking or scratching the treated area. This can cause minor infection, possible scarring and extensive **hyperpigmentation** *(HEYE per pig men TAY shun)*.

UNDERTREATMENT

The most common kind of maltreatment is undertreatment. This occurs when the hair's dermal papillae and surrounding germinative cells have not been totally destroyed and extensive regrowth occurs.

In all acceptable forms of permanent hair removal, the criteria for permanent hair removal is the easy withdrawal of the hair from the treated follicle. If this does not occur after treatment, the hair will simply be tweezed and the hair follicle will grow another hair in its place. The easy release of the hair is not always an indication that the hair follicle is permanently destroyed. Most authorities believe that at least 70% of the tissue should be effectively destroyed. (This will be explained further in Chapter 7.)

Reasons for Undertreatment

There are many reasons for undertreatment. The main reasons are:

1. A heavy-handed technique that would make the practitioner unaware that only simple tweezing is being done.
2. Difficulty in determining easy withdrawal when treating finer hair.
3. Epilator malfunction or when the needle cord or foot pedal are not working properly. The intermittent current would cause many of the hairs to be undertreated or not treated at all.
4. There is a school of thought that believes that the insulated probe does not cause enough germinative tissue damage and therefore causes undertreatment and more regrowth.
5. New devices that are marketed without proper proof of their effectiveness.

SAFEGUARDS FOR EFFECTIVE TREATMENT

Knowledge of the following safeguards will help you give effective treatments to your patients:

1. If the patient feels nothing, then nothing is being accomplished. When tissue is being destroyed, the body must feel it. Make sure the patient can feel the treatment.
2. Validate all new thermolysis epilators with the "bulb test."
3. Remember that all acceptable equipment is either AC or DC. All thermolysis (AC) equipment uses heat to destroy tissue, not electricity. Therefore all equipment of this type produces the same heat patterns.

   All galvanic equipment (DC) produces the same chemical, sodium hydroxide, and will therefore have exactly the same effects on the tissue.

   This also holds true for all dual-method equipment. The only difference would be the sequence of the currents as suggested by the manufacturer or your instructor.

QUESTIONS FOR REVIEW

1. What are 10 causes of overtreatment?
2. What are three factors that could result in undertreatment?
3. What are three safeguards that can help the electrologist ensure that the treatment is adequate?

Chapter 7 Regrowth and Statistics

LEARNING OBJECTIVES
Successful mastery of the material in this chapter will be indicated when you can:

1. Describe the three phases in the life cycle of hair.
2. List regrowth time for hair on various parts of the body.
3. Give at least six regrowth factors.

INTRODUCTION
Patients who seek an electrologist are looking for help. They are unhappy with unwanted hair. The electrologist's function is to make patients happy with themselves. This can only happen if the treatments are successful. Unsuccessful treatments will cause the patient to become anxious and irritable.

When patients have several hours of treatment and still see hair, they can become very upset. They may lose confidence and stop the treatments. This is why the electrologist must be equipped with knowledge of hair growth patterns. The practitioner must adequately explain to the patient in layman's terms the necessity of a schedule of treatments, and the likelihood of follow-ups.

If the patient does not fully understand what is happening, he or she will soon lose confidence and stop the treatments. The electrologist must therefore be able to understand and solve these problems.

HAIR GROWTH CYCLE
Patients may believe that the hair they can see is all they will ever have. They may also believe that what they tweeze today will grow in by tomorrow morning.

All hair goes through a life cycle timed by genes. This cycle can vary from a few months for an eyebrow hair to up to six years or even more for a scalp hair.

The life cycle of a hair begins when a new dermal papilla is formed at the base of the follicle. This begins the *anagen (AN ah jen)* phase. Within a few weeks, a new hair will begin to grow. The early anagen phase continues until the hair is fully grown into a *terminal (TUR mi nal)* or later anagen hair. The *catagen (KAT ah jen)* phase begins when the hair detaches itself from the dermal papilla and for a short period of time receives nourishment from the surrounding network of capillaries. When the hair receives no further nourishment, it is in its *telogen (TEL oh jen)* phase. The dermal papilla and a major portion of the hair follicle shrink considerably. The hair is held within the follicle as a "bed" or "club" hair. These hairs fall out daily through combing, brushing and simple friction.

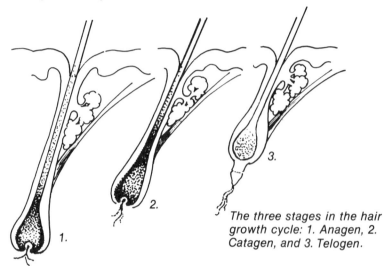

The three stages in the hair growth cycle: 1. Anagen, 2. Catagen, and 3. Telogen.

The time from the anagen to the telogen stages varies depending on the area of the body and the genetic patterns of the patient. Sometimes an early anagen hair will begin to grow before the telogen hair has fallen out. If only the telogen hair is treated, regrowth will occur.

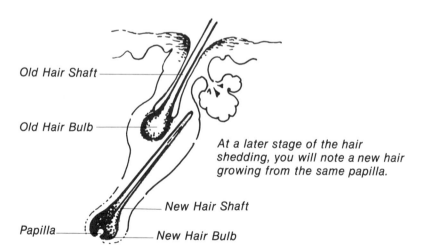

Old Hair Shaft

Old Hair Bulb

At a later stage of the hair shedding, you will note a new hair growing from the same papilla.

New Hair Shaft

Papilla

New Hair Bulb

It is therefore important to know at what rate hair on different parts of the body will regrow after treatment.

Hairs that grow in treated areas before the normal regrowth time are hairs growing from untreated follicles. They are latent (previously dormant) or early anagen hairs.

The following chart details standard regrowth times for vellus and terminal hair on various parts of the body:

REGROWTH TIME CHART	KEY F = female M = male	
Type of Hair		Regrowth Time
Hairline (front or back)	F/M	5 to 6 weeks
Eyebrows	F/M	5 to 6 weeks
Top of nose	F/M	10 to 12 weeks
Upper lip (vellus hair)	F	8 to 9 weeks
Upper lip (terminal)	F/M	4 to 6 weeks
Side of face (vellus)	F	12 to 14 weeks
Side of face (terminal)	F/M	5 to 6 weeks
Chin (vellus)	F	6 to 7 weeks
Chin (terminal)	F/M	5 to 6 weeks
Neck (terminal)	F	5 to 6 weeks
Neck (terminal)	M	4 to 5 weeks
Ears (outside vellus)	F/M	10 to 11 weeks
Ears (outside terminal)	F/M	7 to 8 weeks
Breast	F	7 to 8 weeks
Chest (terminal)	F	7 to 8 weeks
Chest (terminal)	M	6 to 7 weeks
Back & shoulders (terminal)	F	7 to 8 weeks
Back & shoulders (terminal)	M	6 to 7 weeks
Arms (terminal)	F/M	7 to 8 weeks
Legs (terminal)	F/M	6 to 7 weeks
Hands (terminal)	F/M	7 to 8 weeks
Underarms (terminal)	F/M	7 to 8 weeks
Abdomen (terminal)	F	8 to 9 weeks
Inner thighs (terminal)	F	5 to 6 weeks
Feet, toes (terminal)	F/M	6 to 8 weeks

Any hair that appears before the estimated aftertreatment times indicated on this chart is growing from untreated follicles. Patients must understand this or they will blame the electrologist for poor treatment or feel that electrolysis does not work.

These latent early anagen hairs are one of the reasons why patients think treated hair is regrowing. Latent early anagen hairs account for the largest percentage of the "regrowth problem."

Another factor is distorted hair. These are follicles that do not grow straight, but curl under the skin in such a way that a straight needle cannot possibly reach the papilla. Distorted hair follicles occur mostly in patients with curly hair. Sometimes follicles become distorted and thickened from constant tweezing or waxing.

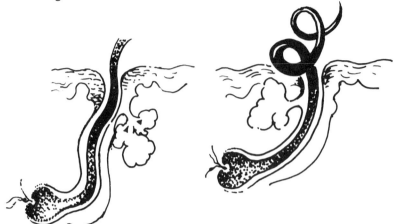

Two examples of distorted follicles.

The average patient has few distorted hairs. *All hairs in the very early anagen stage are straight and lie close to the surface of the skin.* This is the main reason why patients should keep their treatments on a close schedule. In other words, treating a hair in the very early anagen stage assures no distortion. The dermal papilla and hair have not fully matured at this stage, and destruction of these cells at this time is more advantageous. It also requires less needle intensity and depth, which decreases the pain level and after effects.

There will be times when a treated hair will not easily slip out, even with three or four surges of intensity. Simply tweeze the hair. Don't overtreat the area or scarring could occur. This particular hair is usually a distorted hair and so should be treated at a later time when the hair is in early anagen stage.

Many patients who receive treatment have high levels of androgen hormone, which increases the amount of hair and speeds the hair cycle. It is not uncommon for a patient to believe that electrolysis treatments are causing new hair growth. Before treatment, explain that their excessive glandular secretions are causing new hair growth in surrounding follicles. This is especially true if the hair appears in five weeks or less.

If a female patient is growing excessive hair on the lip, chin, neck, breast, abdomen, and inner thighs, she probably has a hormone disorder and an irregular menstrual cycle. This patient should be referred to a physician for treatment. Otherwise these areas will continue to grow hair until all of the follicles in that area are destroyed. Excess hair growth due to hormonal causes can often be reduced by medical treatment. The hair already present, however, must be treated.

It is important to note that each area of the body has a set amount of hair follicles from birth. Most hair follicles are dormant or grow hair that is invisible to the human eye. Once a hair follicle is destroyed it can no longer grow another hair. New hair results only if a dormant follicle becomes active. There can be anywhere from 500 to 1000 hair follicles per square inch, depending on the part of the body.

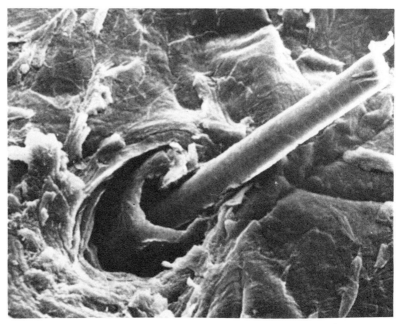

Closeup of a single hair growing from a follicle. There can be anywhere from 500 to 1000 hair follicles per square inch of skin.

REGROWTH PATTERN LIST

A completed area is an area that has been fully cleared and given three months to a year of follow-up treatments.

The areas in the following group tend to grow more new hair as the female patient grows older, especially if there is a genetic or hormonal problem:

The chin
The front area of the neck
The cheeks
The upper lip

Once these areas are completed, however there is less need for follow-up treatments:

The chest (male or female)
The breasts
The ears (male or female)
The back (male)
The top of the nose (male or female)
The feet and toes (female)

Once the following areas are completed, little or no follow-up treatments are necessary. These areas generally grow hair from a set number of hair follicles and rarely grow more than a few new hairs after completion:

The hairline
The eyebrows
The abdomen
The underarms
The arms
The inner thighs
The legs

It is important to know that certain parts of the body tend to grow more new hair than others. With this knowledge, the practitioner can give the patient some idea of future follow-up treatments once an area is completed.

REASONS FOR REGROWTH   Regrowth is defined as hair that regrows from a follicle that has been previously treated.

Undertreatment   Undertreatment means that insufficient energy was used to destroy enough of the dermal papillae and the lower hair follicle so that further growth is prevented.

Poor Insertion   A poor insertion is one in which the electrologist simply misses the target, the papilla. Even if the required intensity and time are used, the hair will regrow.

Distorted Hair Follicles   It is almost impossible to destroy distorted hair with thermolysis except in the early anagen phase of hair growth. Galvanic and blend methods are slightly more effective on distorted hair due to the flow of sodium hydroxide.

Telogen Hair   Most experts agree that hair in the telogen phase of growth has no dermal papillae or germinative cells. Since the dermal papilla must be destroyed before treatment can be permanent, it is not known whether any process of electrology can be effective on hair in this phase.

Bed or Club Hair   Bed or club hair can have another hair in early anagen growing beneath it. The new hair would then emerge aftertreatment, appearing to be regrowth.

Unapproved Methods   The use of devices that have not been proven effective for permanent hair removal can easily cause regrowth.

Apparent Regrowth   Often hair appears to be regrowing when in fact it is growing from adjacent follicles. This occurs when active follicles are especially close together, or when latent or dormant follicles become active.

Two or more hairs can also emerge from a single follicle, and more than one electrology treatment may be necessary when this occurs.

Hormonal disturbances can stimulate the follicles to grow more new hair and at a faster rate. Hormones can also cause vellus hair to grow darker and deeper, becoming terminal hair.

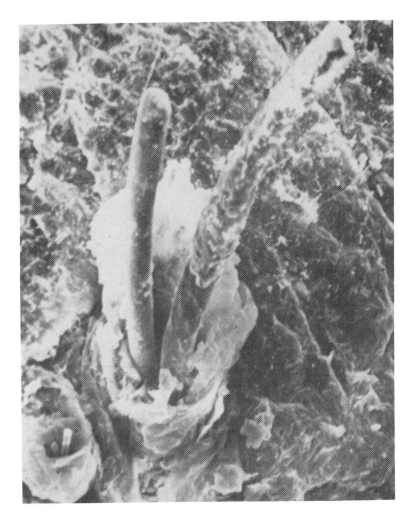

Two or more hairs can emerge from a single follicle, as is illustrated in this photo.

QUESTIONS FOR   1. What are the three phases in the life cycle of hair?
REVIEW   2. What is the regrowth time for hair on each part of the body?
     3. What are at least six regrowth factors?

Chapter 8 Bacteriology

LEARNING OBJECTIVES Successful mastery of the material in this chapter will be indicated when you can:

1. Define bacteria and list two types.
2. Explain bacterial growth and reproduction.
3. List the symptoms of bacterial infections and indicate their importance to electrology.
4. Describe methods for destruction of bacteria.
5. Discuss methods to prevent disease.

INTRODUCTION Ancient people had no knowledge of science and regarded disease as supernatural. They believed their gods sent disease and disaster as punishment. To appease the gods, these ancient people developed rituals they hoped would prevent disease and injury. As civilization progressed, people realized that diseases were contagious and that they were transmitted by clothing and other objects via bacteria. A Dutch naturalist, Anton Van Leeuwenhock (1632-1723), is credited with the discovery of bacteria. He invented a microscope which could magnify up to 300 times. The microscope enabled him to study bacteria, molds, and protozoa.

NOTE: *Bacteriology (bak teer ee OL oh jee)* is the branch of biology that deals with the study of *microorganisms (meye kroh OR ga niz ems).*

The electrologist should first study bacteriology in order to understand the importance of sanitation and sterilization as it applies to the profession. Electrologists must understand how the spread of disease can be prevented, and be aware of the precautions to be taken to protect their own as well as their patients' health. They must understand the relationship of bacteria to the principles of school and office cleanliness and sanitation.

Contagious diseases, skin infections, and blood poisoning are caused either by the passing of infectious material directly from one individual to another, or by unsanitary implements that have been used first on an infected person and then are used on someone else. Other sources of contagion are dirty hands and fingernails, contaminated containers, and unsanitary facilities. Sources of contagion must be eliminated in the professional electrology office, and most states have regulatory agencies that require correct sanitary measures.

THREE GENERAL FORMS OF BACTERIA

Cocci	Bacilli	Spirilla
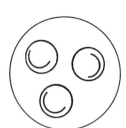	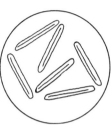	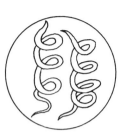

GROUPINGS OF BACTERIA

Diplococci	Streptococci	Staphylococci
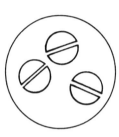	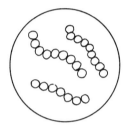	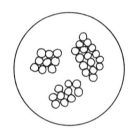

SIX DISEASE PRODUCING BACTERIA

Typhoid Bacillus Showing Flagella	Tubercle Bacillus (Tuberculosis)	Diphtheria Bacillus
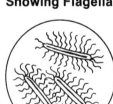	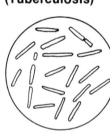	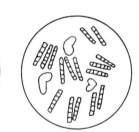

Bacillus Influenza	Cholera (Microspira)	Tetanus Bacillus With Spores
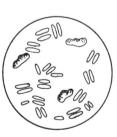	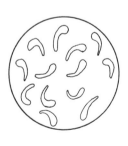	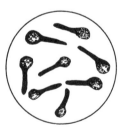

REMINDER   *Although bacteria cannot be seen with the naked eye, it is very important to practice cleanliness and sanitation at all times, to prevent the spread of contagious disease.*

BACTERIA   **Bacteria** are minute, one-celled vegetable microorganisms that are found nearly everywhere. They are especially numerous in dust, dirt, refuse, and diseased tissue. Bacteria are also known as **germs** or **microbes.** Bacteria are especially numerous on the skin of the body and in water, air, decayed matter, bodily secretions, on clothing, and under the free edge of the nails.

Ordinarily, bacteria are not visible except with the aid of a microscope. Fifteen hundred rod-shaped bacteria will barely reach across the head of a pin.

Types of Bacteria   There are hundreds of different kinds of bacteria. These are generally classified into two types, either beneficial (harmless) or disease producing (harmful).

1. **Nonpathogenic** *(NON path o GEN ik)* organisms (beneficial or harmless type) are the majority of all bacteria. They perform many useful functions, such as decomposing refuse and improving the fertility of the soil. To this group belong the **saprophytes** *(SAP ro feyet),* which live on dead matter but do not produce disease.
2. **Pathogenic** *path o GEN ik)* organisms (harmful type), although they are in the minority, cause considerable damage when they invade plant or animal tissue. Pathogenic bacteria are harmful because they produce disease. To this group belong **parasites** *(PAR a seyet),* which require living matter for their growth.

It is because of these pathogenic bacteria that the practice of sterilization and sanitation is especially necessary in a school or office.

Classification of Pathogenic Bacteria   Bacteria show distinct forms of shapes which aid in their identification. We are concerned with pathogenic bacteria, which are classified as follows:

1. **Cocci** *(KOK seye)* are round-shaped organisms which appear singly or in groups. Those which form in groups include:
   a. **Staphylococci** *(STAF i lo KOK seye),* which are pus-forming organisms which grow in bunches or clusters. They are present in abscesses, pustules, and boils.
   b. **Streptococci** *(STREP to KOK seye),* which are pus-forming organisms which grow in chains.
   c. **Diplococci** *(DIP lo KOK seye),* which grow in pairs. They cause pneumonia.
2. **Bacilli** *(BA cil lee)* are rod-shaped organisms which present either a short, thin, or thick structure. They are the most common and produce such diseases as tetanus (lockjaw), influenza, typhoid fever, tuberculosis, and diphtheria. Many bacilli are spore forming.
3. **Spirilla** *(spi RIL ah)* are curved or corkscrew-shaped organisms. They are subdivided into several groups.

BACTERIAL GROWTH AND REPRODUCTION

Bacteria are composed of an outer cell membrane and an internal protoplasm. They manufacture their own food from the surrounding environment, give off waste products, grow and reproduce.

Bacteria exhibit two distinct phases in their life cycle: The active or **vegetative** stage, and the inactive or **spore-forming** stage.

Active or Vegetative Bacteria

During the active stage, bacteria grow and reproduce. Microorganisms multiply best in warm, dark, damp, dirty places, where sufficient food is present.

When conditions are favorable, bacteria reproduce very quickly. As food is absorbed, the bacterial cell grows in size. When the limit of growth is reached, the bacterial cell divides crosswise into halves, thereby forming two daughter cells. From one original bacterium, as many as 16 million germs may develop in half a day.

When favorable conditions cease to exist, bacteria either die or become inactive.

Inactive or Spore-Forming Bacteria

Certain bacteria (such as the anthrax and tetanus bacilli), form **spores** in order to withstand periods of famine, drought, and unsuitable temperature. In this stage, spores can be blown about in the dust and not be harmed by disinfectants, heat, or cold.

When favorable conditions are restored, the spores enter the active or vegetative stage, and start to grow and reproduce.

Movement of Bacteria

For the most part, only the bacilli and spirilla are able to move about. The cocci rarely show mobility. Bacteria move by means of hairlike projections, known as **flagella** *(fla **GEL** la)* or **cilia** *(SIL ee ah)*. The movement of these hairs propels the bacteria about in liquid.

BACTERIAL INFECTIONS

Pathogenic bacteria become a menace when they invade the body. An infection occurs if the body is unable to cope with the bacteria and the harmful toxins they produce. A local infection is indicated by a boil or a pimple containing pus.

A general infection results when the blood stream carries the bacteria and their toxins to all parts of the body, as in blood poisoning.

The electrologist's needle can be a means used by bacteria to invade the body. Sterilization of the needle before treatment is the best means of prevention.

Pus

The presence of pus is a sign of infection. Staphylococci are the most common pus-forming bacteria. Found in pus are bacteria, waste matter, decayed tissue, body cells, and blood cells.

Contagious Disease

A disease becomes contagious, or communicable, when it spreads from one person to another by contact. Some of the more common contagious diseases which would prevent an electrologist from working are tuberculosis, ringworm, scabies, lice, viral infections, and any type of skin disease.

Sources of Infection   The chief sources of infection are unclean hands and instruments, open sores, mouth and nose discharges, and the common use of drinking cups and towels. Coughing, sneezing, and spitting also spread germs.

Through personal hygiene and public sanitation, infections can be prevented and controlled.

 CAUTION: *An electrologist should never treat a patient who has hemophilia, open sores, or a bacterial infection of the heart. This is because the skin heals through the formation of scabs after an electrology treatment. A patient with any of these conditions will have difficulty healing, and may be prone to infection or other complications.*

Bacterial Entry   There can be no infection without the presence of a pathogenic agent. Pathogenic bacteria may enter the body by way of:

1. A break in the skin, such as a cut, pimple, or scratch.
2. Breathing (air) or swallowing (water or food).
3. The nose (air).
4. The eyes or ears (dirt.)
5. Sexual contact.

Body Defenses   The body fights infection by means of its defensive forces such as:

1. The unbroken skin (the body's first defense).
2. Body secretions, such as perspiration and digestive juices.
3. White blood cells.
4. Antitoxins which counteract the toxins produced by bacteria.

Other Infectious Agents   **Filterable viruses** are living organisms so small that they will pass through the pores of a porcelain filter. They cause the common cold and other **respiratory** *(RES pi ra tohr ee)* and **gastrointestinal** *(gas troh in TES ti nal)* infections.

Parasites are plants or animals which live upon other living organisms without giving anything in return.

Plant parasites or **fungi** *(FUN jee)*, such as molds, mildews, and yeasts, can produce such contagious diseases as ringworm and favus.

Animal parasites, such as certain insects, are responsible for such contagious diseases as scabies, due to the itch mite, and **pediculosis** *(pe DIK yoo LOH sis)*, caused by lice.

 CAUTION: *Contagious diseases caused by parasites should never be treated in a school or office. Patients should be referred to their physician.*

Immunity

Immunity *(i MYOO ni tee)* is the ability of the body to resist invasion by bacteria or to destroy bacteria after entry. Immunity to disease is a sign of good health. It may be natural or acquired. Natural immunity means resistance to disease from birth, which can be maximized by hygienic living. Acquired immunity occurs after the body has overcome diseases, or after it has received vaccinations.

Acquired Immune Deficiency Syndrome

Acquired Immune Deficiency Syndrome (AIDS) should not cause excessive concern to the electrologist. Proper sterilization of needles between patients will prevent contamination. This can be done with the autoclave.

Some electrologists prefer the use of disposable needles for each patient. As an alternative, the patient may choose to buy a needle and bring it for each treatment.

Human Disease Carrier

A **human disease carrier** is a person who is immune to a disease, and yet carries germs that can infect other people. **Typhoid** *(TEYE foid)* fever and **diphtheria** *(dip THEER ee a)* may be transmitted in this manner.

DESTRUCTION OF BACTERIA

Bacteria may be destroyed by exposure to disinfectants, intense heat (such as that produced by the autoclave or glass bead sterilizer) and ultra-violet rays.

Vaccinations

Vaccinations are effective against such diseases as polio, typhoid fever, chicken pox, smallpox, whooping cough, measles, tetanus, and other diseases.

Antibiotics

Antibiotics *(an ti beye OT iks)* are substances that destroy an organism or inhibit its growth. Antibiotics are produced by various microorganisms and fungi. They have the power to slow growth and to destroy other microorganisms. **Penicillin** is an antibiotic produced in several forms for the treatment of a wide variety of bacterial infections. Many electrologists recommend that their patients use an antibacterial cream after treatment.

Body Defenses

The body is constantly defending itself against invasion by disease. Its defenses are called *first-, second-,* and *third-line* defenses.

First-Line Defenses

Bacteria can enter the body through any opening, such as the mouth, nose, and so forth. Bacteria are taken into the body in food and liquids, or can enter by way of breaks, cuts, or punctures in the skin.

Healthy skin is one of the body's most important defenses against disease. It acts as a barrier by resisting the penetration of harmful bacteria.

The nose has mucus and fine hairs that serve as protection against bacteria. A sneeze or cough, for example, is the body protecting itself against bacteria. Other barriers are created by mucus membranes in the mouth, gastric juices in the stomach, and organisms within the intestines and other areas of the body. Tears in the eyes also serve to flush out harmful bacteria and foreign objects.

 CAUTION: *The electrologist should never treat the hair inside the nose. This can cause serious infection and possible death.*

Second-Line Defenses   The body also defends itself from harmful bacteria by producing **inflammation** *(in fla MAY* shun). Redness and swelling indicate an increase in temperature and metabolic activity. The inflamed area will be sensitive to the touch. The **white corpuscles** go into action to destroy harmful microorganisms in the bloodstream so that healing can take place.

Third-Line Defenses   The body can produce substances which inhibit or destroy harmful bacteria. These protective substances are called **antibodies.**

PREVENTION OF DISEASE   To avoid the spread of disease, keep yourself and your surroundings sanitary. Keep everything you touch clean. Check that everything you use is clean before use, and sanitized afterward. You must be aware of the importance of personal hygienic living, which includes eating healthful and nourishing foods, getting proper rest and exercise, and having regular physical check-ups in order to maintain your health.

Refuse to treat any person who has a contagious disease or infection, and you should suggest, tactfully, that the patient see a physician.

QUESTIONS FOR REVIEW
1. What are bacteria? Name and briefly describe two types.
2. How do bacteria grow and reproduce?
3. What are the symptoms of bacterial infections? Why is it important that the electrologist recognize infection?
4. How can bacteria be destroyed?
5. How can disease be prevented?

Chapter 9 Sterilization and Sanitation

LEARNING OBJECTIVES

Successful mastery of the material in this chapter will be indicated when you can:

1. Explain the structure and functions of the autoclave.
2. Describe four types of chemical disinfectant agents used in the electrology office.
3. List six safety precautions related to sterilization and sanitation.
4. Define the terms "sterilize" and "sanitize."
5. Give twenty rules of sanitation.

INTRODUCTION

Sterilization is the process of making an object germ-free. It involves destroying all pathogenic (infectious) bacteria, as well as all nonpathogenic bacteria, which are not harmful.

Sterilization is of practical importance to the electrologist because it deals with methods used either to prevent the growth of germs or to destroy them entirely. It is especially important to destroy those microorganisms that are responsible for infectious and communicable diseases.

Health departments and other governmental agencies recognize that it is impossible to maintain as sterile an environment as is found in hospitals, but require that you sterilize instruments and follow strict sanitation procedures in the school and office. The office and school work areas, all implements and equipment, and the dispensary must be kept in sanitary condition at all times.

METHODS OF STERILIZATION AND SANITATION

There are five well known methods of sterilization and sanitation. These are grouped under two main headings: *physical agents* and *chemical agents.*

Physical Agents

Steaming through the use of an autoclave is one of the most effective methods of sterilization in the practice of electrology. It is recommended for sterilizing needles, which are reused from patient to patient. Some professionals feel that **glass bead sterilizing** is also effective for sterilizing needles.

Boiling objects in water at 212°F (100°C) for 20 minutes will achieve sterilization. In general, schools and electrology offices no longer use this method because it is time-consuming and may damage certain objects.

Dry heat is a method of sterilization often used in hospitals to sterilize bedding and similar materials.

Ultraviolet rays destroy most bacteria. Ultraviolet rays in an electrical sanitizer are used in schools and offices to keep sanitized instruments sanitary.

NOTE: *Though several methods of sterilization are listed, electrologists commonly wash instruments with soap and water and wipe with alcohol to sanitize (i.e., retard or kill bacteria present) them. The exception is the needle, which is always sterilized.*

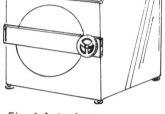

Sterilizers. An important piece of sterilizing equipment is the autoclave. The **autoclave** (Fig. 1) is an airtight chamber which fills with pressurized steam at a temperature of between 240° and 254°F. The steam effectively sterilizes instruments left in the chamber for 15 minutes or longer.

Fig. 1 Autoclave

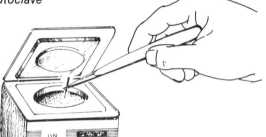

The sterilization capacity of the glass bead sterilizer is an area of controversy among experts.

Another method of sterilization used by some electrologists is the **glass bead sterilizer** (Fig. 2). It contains a chamber inside of which rests a colander-like container filled with glass beads. Needles are placed inside the glass beads, which are then heated to between 500° and 800°F. The sterilization capacity of the glass bead sterilizer is an area of controversy among experts. Some professionals feel that leaving needles inside the glass bead sterilizer for a period of 24 hours will ensure sterilization. Others feel that only needles which have previously been washed and then sterilized in an autoclave should be placed in a glass bead sterilizer (in effect, using the glass bead sterilizer to *maintain* a state of sterilization). Be guided by your instructor in this matter.

Fig. 2 Glass bead sterilizer.

Chemical Agents

Various types of chemical agents are used for sanitizing purposes. These are antiseptics, and disinfectants (germicides).

An **antiseptic** is a substance which will retard the growth of bacteria. Antiseptics are generally milder than disinfectants, and are safer to use on the skin.

Some soaps are beneficial as antiseptics when used to wash the hands and implements. However, soap and water alone are not enough to thoroughly sanitize the hands or implements. General antiseptics include alcohol, hydrogen peroxide, formaldehyde, and chlorine bleach. These substances should be used as recommended by the manufacturers. Refer to the chart included in this chapter for names, forms, strengths, and uses of various antiseptics.

A **disinfectant** is stronger than an antiseptic and must be used with caution. Chemical agents are classified as strong solutions (those used as disinfectants), and weaker solutions (those used as antiseptics).

Refer to the chart included in this chapter for names, forms, strengths, and uses of various disinfectants. Other approved antiseptics and disinfectants are used in electrology offices. Consult the regulatory agency in your state which regulates electrology for their recommendations.

Requirements of a Good Disinfectant

A good disinfectant must be:

1. Convenient to prepare.
2. Fast Acting.
3. Preferably odorless.
4. Noncorrosive.
5. Economical.
6. Nonirritating to skin.

Types of Disinfectant

There are many chemical disinfectant agents on the market which are sold ready for use. If these are used, select the ones that have been approved by the regulatory agency in your state. Chemicals commonly used in the office are:

1. **Quaternary ammonium compounds** ("quats")—used to sanitize implements.
2. **Formaldehyde**—used to sanitize implements, and to maintain dry sanitizers.
3. **Alcohol**—used to sanitize instruments.
4. **Prepared products**—used to clean floors, sinks, and toilet bowls.

Chemical Sanitizing Agents "Quats"

Quaternary ammonium compounds *(KWAH ter nah ree ah MOH nee um CAHM pownds)* or "quats" are a broad range of surface-active chemical agents of importance in the office. Quats are formulated into products that you will use as disinfectants, cleansers, sterilizers, and fungicides for sanitation purposes that we will discuss in this chapter.

The advantages claimed for quats as sanitation agents are that they offer a short disinfection time, and are odorless, colorless, nontoxic, and stable. Immersion time ranges from 1 to 5 minutes, depending on the strength of the solution used.

CAUTION:

*Before using any sanitizing agent, read and follow manufacturer's directions on label and any accompanying literature. Find out if the product can be used on naturally soft or hard water or water that has been softened. Inquire whether it contains a rust inhibitor. Should the product lack a rust inhibitor, the additon of ½% **sodium nitrite** (SOH dee um **NEYE** trayt) to the solution prevents the rusting of metallic implements.*

SOLUTION STRENGTHS

How to prepare a 1:1000 strength solution of quaternary ammonium compound.

10% active ingredient	Add 1¼ oz. (37.5 ml) quat solution to 1 gal. (3.8 l) of water.
12% active ingredient	Add 1 oz. (30 ml) quat solution to 1 gal. (3.8 l) of water.
15% active ingredient	Add ¾ oz. (22.5 ml) quat solution to 1 gal (3.8 l) of water.

Formaldehyde. **Formaldehyde** *(for MAL de heyed)* is an effective sanitizing agent which can be used as a disinfectant. As purchased, Formalin is approximately 37% to 40% formaldehyde gas in water. Formalin should be used with great care as inhalation can cause damage to mucous membranes and contact with the skin can cause irritation. Due to its potential dangers, Formalin is most commonly added to prepared sanitizing agents and used in various strengths as follows: A 25% solution is used to sanitize implements. Immerse them for at least 10 minutes. A 10% solution may be used to maintain previously sanitized instruments. A 5% formaldehyde solution may be used as a disinfectant to immerse instruments in. A 2% solution may be used as an antiseptic for small areas of skin.

Alcohol. **Alcohol** is sold in different strengths. 70% alcohol acts as a disinfectant and 30% to 40% alcohol acts as an antiseptic. An advantage of alcohol is that it dissolves dirt and makeup and will not corrode or discolor instruments.

The following is an easy reference chart of the disinfectants and antiseptics used in the electrology office.

DISINFECTANTS USED IN OFFICES:

Name	Form	Strength	Uses
Quaternary ammonium compounds ("quats")	Liquid or tablet	1:1000 solution	Immerse implements in solution for 1 to 5 minutes.
Formalin	Liquid	25% solution	Immerse implements in solution for 10 minutes.
Formalin	Liquid	10% solution	Immerse implements in solution for 20 minutes.
Ethyl or grain alcohol	Liquid	70% solution	Sanitize sharp cutting implements and electrodes.
Cresol (Lysol)	Liquid	10% soap solution	Cleanse floors, sinks, and toilets.

ANTISEPTICS USED IN OFFICES:

Name	Form	Strength	Uses
Boric acid	White crystals	2-5% solution	Cleanse the eyes
Tincture of iodine	Liquid	2% solution	Cleanse cuts and wounds.
Hydrogen peroxide	Liquid	3% solution	Cleanse skin and minor cuts.
Ethyl or grain alcohol	Liquid	60% solution	Cleanse hands, skin and minute cuts. Not to be used if irritation is present.
Chloramine—T (Chlorazene: Chlorozol)	White crystals	½% solution	Cleanse skin and hands and for general use.
Sodium Hypochlorite	White crystals	½% solution	Rinse the hands.

NOTE: *Other approved disinfectants and antiseptics may be used in the electrology office. Consult with the regulatory agency in your state as well as with your instructor.*

SAFETY PRECAUTIONS

1. Purchase chemicals in small quantities and store them in a cool, dry place; otherwise, they deteriorate due to contact with air, light, and heat.
2. Weigh and measure chemicals carefully.
3. Keep all containers labeled.
4. Read all labels and follow directions carefully.
5. Do not breathe fumes from chemicals or solutions.
6. Avoid spilling when diluting chemicals.
7. When performing a service, make sure your hands have been washed and sanitized.
8. Make sure that the work area and all materials and equipment used are either sanitized or sterilized.
9. Keep all products organized in order to prevent accidental spills and breakage.
10. To avoid contamination, never use fingers to remove a product from a container. Use a sanitized spatula or sterile cotton.
11. Always keep antiseptics and disinfectants sealed and in a safe place. They should always be clearly labeled and never transferred to unlabeled containers where they may be mistaken for some other product.

**DEFINITIONS
PERTAINING TO
SANITATION**

1. **Sterilize** *(STER i leyez)*—to render sterile; to make free from all bacteria (harmful or beneficial) by the act of sterilizing.
2. **Sterile** *(STER il)*—free from all germs.
3. **Antiseptic** *(an ti SEP tik)*—a chemical agent which may kill or retard the growth of bacteria.
4. **Disinfect** *(dis in FEKT)*—to destroy bacteria on any object.
5. **Disinfectant** *(dis in FEK tant)*—a chemical agent having the power to destroy bacteria (germs or microbes).
6. **Bactericide** *(bak TEER i seyed)*—a chemical agent having the power to destroy bacteria (germs of microbes).
7. **Germicide** *(JUR mi seyed)*—a chemical agent having the power to destroy germs.
8. **Asepsis** *(ay SEP sis)*—freedom from disease causing germs.
9. **Sepsis** *(SEP sis)*—poisoning due to pathogenic bacteria.
10. **Fumigant** *(FYOO mi gant)*—vapor used to keep clean objects sanitary.
11. **Sanitize** *(SAN i teyez)*S to render objects clean and relatively germ free.

SANITATION

Sanitation is the application of measures to promote public health and prevent the spread of infectious diseases. The importance of sanitation cannot be overemphasized. Electrology brings the electrologist in direct contact with the patient's skin. Understanding sanitary measures contributes to the protection of the patient's health.

Various governmental agencies protect community health by providing for a wholesome food and water supply and quick disposal of refuse. These steps are only a few of the ways in which the public health is safeguarded.

**Sanitation and the
Office Environment**

The air within an electrology office should be neither dry nor stagnant, nor have a stale, musty odor. Room temperature should be about 70° F.

The office can also be ventilated with the aid of an exhaust fan or an air conditioner. Air conditioning has the advantage of permitting changes in the quality and quantity of air brought into the office. The temperature and moisture content of the air can also be regulated by means of air conditioning.

Drinking water should be odorless, colorless, and free from any foreign matter. Crystal clear water may still be unsanitary because of the presence of pathogenic bacteria which cannot be seen with the naked eye.

Infected Patients

A patient who has an infectious disease is of course contagious to others. Electrologists who have colds or other communicable disease must not be permitted to treat patients. Likewise, patients obviously suffering from an infectious disease must not be accommodated in the electrology office. In this way, the best interest of other patients will be served. The State Board of Cosmetology and Board of Health in many states or localities have formulated sanitary regulations which apply to the practice of electrology.

NOTE: *Patients suffering from acquired immune deficiency syndrome (AIDS), herpes, or other sexually transmitted diseases (STDs) should be treated with great caution. NEVER place a needle near an open sore. Needles used to treat patients with STDs should be sterilized afterward in either a glass bead sterilizer or a dry or wet steam autoclave. Be advised by your instructor in this matter. Another alternative when treating patients with STDs is to use disposable needles.*

Rules of Sanitation

Following these rules will result in cleaner and safer service to the public:

1. Chemical solutions in sanitizers should be changed as often as necessary.
2. Implements should be kept in a disinfectant solution (70% alcohol) until ready for use.
3. All implements that are used more than once must be sanitized after each patient. *NEEDLES MUST BE STERILIZED.*
4. All implements must be placed on a sanitary surface or in sanitary containers while not in use.
5. All trays and other items must be sanitized before and after each patient.
6. All appliances should be sanitized after each patient by swabbing with sterile cotton dampened with 70% alcohol or other solution recommended by your instructor for this purpose.
7. The practice of immersing implements in a chemical solution should conform to regulations issued by your state.
8. Every office must be well lit, and heated or cooled as patient need demands.
9. The office should be properly ventilated and clean.
10. The walls, curtains, floor, and floor coverings in an electrology office should be washable and, they should always be clean.
11. All offices must be supplied with continuous hot and cold running water. Drinking facilities (individual cups and a water cooler and/or fountain) should be provided.
12. All plumbing fixtures should be properly installed.
13. The premises should be kept free of rodents and insects.
14. The office should never be used for cooking, sleeping, or living quarters.
15. Any waste material dropped on the floor must be removed from the floor without delay and deposited in closed containers. Remove such materials from the premises at frequent intervals.
16. Rest rooms must be kept in a sanitary condition and provided with hot and cold running water, liquid soap, paper towels, and toilet paper.
17. Each electrologist must wear a clean, washable uniform while working on patients.
18. The electrologist must cleanse his or her hands thoroughly before and after treating each patient and after using the rest room.

19. Freshy laundered towels or paper towels must be used for each patient. Towels that are ready for use must be stored in clean, closed closets.
20. A clean towel should be placed on the headrest for each patient.
21. Creams and ointments used must be kept in clean, closed containers. Spatulas, not fingers, must be used for removing cream from jars. Sterile cotton or cosmetic sponges may be used to apply lotions and powders. Jars and bottles should be covered when not in use.
22. All soiled and used items must be removed from the area immediately after use. Never mix used items with sanitized, unused items.
23. Never place any item in your mouth or in your pocket.
24. Never allow patients to wear gowns or headbands that have been worn by another patient.
25. All implements and articles used when giving a treatment must be washed, sanitized, and placed in an airtight container or a cabinet sterilizer.
26. The electrologist must refrain from touching his or her face or hair while treating a patient. If it is necessary to do so, the hands must be sanitized again before touching the patient or before handling any of the implements or articles being used for treatment.
27. No pets of any type can be permitted in an office or school.

REMINDERS: *The responsibility for sanitation rests with each student in the school, and with each electrologist in the office. The owner must provide the necessities for school and office sanitation.*

The electrologist must obey the rules of sanitation issued by the agency that regulates electrology treatment regarding acceptable sanitation methods.

QUESTIONS FOR REWIEW:
1. What are the structures and functions of the autoclave?
2. What are four chemical disinfectant agents used in the electrology office? How are they used?
3. What are six safety precautions related to sterilization and sanitation?
4. What are the definitions for "sterilize" and "sanitize"?
5. What are the twenty rules of sanitation?

Chapter 10 Cells, Metabolism, and Body Systems

LEARNING OBJECTIVES

Successful mastery of the material in this chapter will be indicated when you can:

1. Define a cell.
2. Describe the structure of the cell.
3. List the nine systems of the body.

INTRODUCTION

It is important for the electrologist to have a thorough understanding of the health, growth, repair, and functions of the skin. It is therefore necessary for electrologists to study the major parts of the body to be treated.

The body is composed of **cells, tissues, organs,** and **systems.** It is made up of one-fourth solid matter and three-fourths liquid. The human body develops from a single cell. Cells have different functions that include the movements of substances through the cell membranes, reproduction, and metabolism. Cells reproduce themselves by dividing, and groups of cells form the body tissues which become the organs that make up the various systems of the body. The skin is made up of membrane-like tissue covering the entire body.

CELLS

The **cell** is the basic unit of all living things. Every part of the body is composed of cells, which differ from each other in size, shape, structure, and function.

A cell is a minute portion of living substance containing **protoplasm (PROH to plaz em)**, which is colorless, jelly-like matter containing food elements and water.

STRUCTURE OF THE CELL

The protoplasm of the cell contains the following structures:

Nucleus (NOO kli us)—dense protoplasm found in the cell's center, which plays an important role in cell reproduction.

Cytoplasm (SEYE to plaz em)—less dense protoplasm found outside the nucleus, which contains food necessary for the growth, reproduction, and repair of the cell.

Centrosome (SEN troh sohm)—a small, round body in the cytoplasm, which also affects the reproduction of the cell.

Cell membrane—encloses the protoplasm and permits soluble substances to enter and leave the cell.

Structure of the Cell

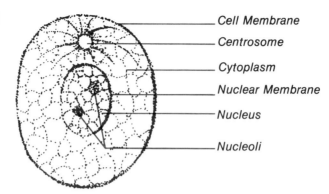

Cell Membrane
Centrosome
Cytoplasm
Nuclear Membrane
Nucleus
Nucleoli

Indirect Division

The division of the human cell is a complex process. It begins with a series of changes that occur in the nucleus before the cell divides in half. The centrosome plays an important role in this procedure, helping to maintain the characteristics of the original cell. This method of reproduction occurs in all human tissues, including hair and skin. This process of reproduction is known as **mitosis** *(meye TOH sis).*

Cell Growth and Reproduction

As long as the cell receives an adequate supply of food, oxygen, and water, eliminates waste products, and is favored with proper temperature, it will continue to grow and thrive. However, if these requirements are not fulfilled, and the presence of **toxins** (poisons) or pressure is evident, then the growth and the health of the cell is impaired. Most body cells are capable of growth and self-repair during their life cycle. *It is the function of electrolysis treatment to prevent new production of cells in the dermal papilla and surrounding germinative cells.*

When a human cell reaches maturity, reproduction takes place by **indirect division.** In this process, a series of changes occur in the nucleus before the entire cell divides in half. Remember that the nucleus is surrounded by a thinner form of protoplasm, called cytoplasm, which supplies the food materials necessary for growth and reproduction.

Indirect Division of a Cell

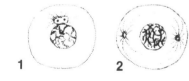

1   2   3   4   5   6

Metabolism

Metabolism *(me TAB o liz em)* is a complex chemical process whereby the body cells are nourished and supplied with the energy they need to carry on their activities.

There are two phases of metabolism:

1. **Anabolism** *(ah NAB o liz em)*—the building up of cellular tissues. During anabolism, the cells of the body absorb water, food, and oxygen for the purposes of growth, reproduction, and repair.

2. **Catabolism** *(ka TAB o liz em)*—the breaking down of cellular tissues. During catabolism, the cells consume what they have absorbed in order to perform specialized functions, such as muscular effort, secretions, or digestion.

Cells have various duties. They make up and renew all parts of the body. They assist in blood circulation by carrying food to the blood and waste matter from the blood. They control all bodily functions.

Tissues

Tissues are composed of groups of cells of the same type. Each tissue has a specific function and can be recognized by its characteristic appearance. Body tissues are classified as follows:

- **Connective tissue** serves to support, protect, and bind together other tissues of the body. Bone, cartilage, ligament, tendon, and fat tissue are examples of connective tissue.
- **Muscular tissue** contracts and moves in various parts of the body.
- **Nerve tissue** carries messages to and from the brain and controls and coordinates all body functions.
- **Epithelial** *(ep i THEE li al)* tissue is a protective covering on body surfaces, such as the skin, mucous membranes, and linings of the heart, digestive and respiratory organs, and glands.
- **Liquid tissue** (blood and lymph) carries food, waste products, and hormones.

Organs

Organs are structures containing two or more different tissues which are combined to accomplish a specific function.

The most important organs of the body are: the brain, which controls the body; the heart, which circulates the blood; the liver, which removes the toxic products of digestion; the kidneys, which excrete water and other waste products; the stomach and intestines, which digest food; and, of special importance to the electrologist, the skin. The skin protects the body, regulates body heat, excretes perspiration and responds to sensation. For further information on the skin see chapter 14.

SYSTEMS

Systems are groups of organs that cooperate for a common purpose, namely the welfare of the entire body. The human body is composed of the following important systems:

Skeletal *(SKEL e tal)* system—bones.
Muscular *(MUS kyu lar)* system—muscles.
Nervous *(NUR vus)* system—nerves.
Circulatory *(SUR kyu la tohr ee)* system—blood supply.
Endocrine *(EN do krin)* system—ductless glands.
Excretory *(EK skre tohr ee)* system—organs of elimination.
Respiratory *(RES pi ra tohr ee)* system—lungs.
Digestive *(di GEST tiv)* system—stomach and intestines.
Reproductive *(re pro DUK tiv)* system—reproduction.

Skeletal System   This is the physical foundation or framework of the body. The function of the **skeletal system** is to serve as a means of protection, support, and locomotion.

Muscular System   The **muscular system** covers, shapes, and supports the skeleton. Its function is to produce all the movements of the body.

Nervous System   The **nervous system** controls and coordinates the functions of all the other systems and makes them work harmoniously and efficiently.

Circulatory System   The circulatory system consists of a closed system of vessels, such as arteries, veins, and capillaries, which carry blood from the heart to all parts of the body, and then back to the heart. This system supplies body cells with food materials, and also carries away waste products.

Endocrine System   The **endocrine system** is composed of a group of specialized glands, which can either benefit or adversely affect the growth, reproduction, health of the body, and is directly and indirectly responsible for all hair growth.

Excretory System   The **excretory system,** which includes the kidneys, liver, skin, intestines, and lungs, purifies the body by eliminating waste products.

Respiratory System   The **respiratory system,** whose most important organs are the trachea (windpipe), bronchial tubes, and lungs, supplies the body with oxygen and removes carbon dioxide.

Digestive System   The **digestive system** changes food into soluble form, suitable for use by the cells of the body.

Reproductive System   The **reproductive system** performs the function of reproducing and perpetuating the human race. This system is related to the endocrine system and therefore affects hair growth

NOTE: *All these systems are closely interrelated and dependent upon each other. While each forms a unit specially designed to perform a specific function, that function cannot be performed without the complete cooperation of some other system or systems. Of all the body systems, the endocrine system is the most important to the electrologist.*

QUESTIONS FOR REVIEW
1. What is a cell?
2. Name the main structures found In the cell.
3. What are the nine systems of the body?

Chapter 11 Human Anatomy

LEARNING OBJECTIVES

Successful mastery of the material in this chapter will be indicated when you can:

1. Give the functions of the bones.
2. List the three kinds of muscular tissue and specify where in the body each can be found.
3. List the divisions of the nervous system and explain the function of each division.
4. Give the two systems of blood circulation and explain how they work.
5. Explain the functions of glands.
6. Give the importance of the excretory system.
7. Describe the composition of the lungs.
8. Explain the function of the digestive system.

INTRODUCTION

The electrologist is not expected to be an anatomy expert, but it is important for him or her to understand the structure of the areas being treated.

Anatomy *(ah NAHT o mee)* is the study of the organs and systems of the body, such as muscles, bones, and arteries. The electrologist is concerned with the body parts treated in the office, such as the face, neck, legs, and arms.

Histology *(hi STOL o jee)* is the study of the minute structures of the body. The electrologist is particularly concerned with the histology of the skin and its appendages; that is, hair, nails, and sweat and oil glands.

Physiology *(fiz i OL o jee)* is the study of the functions or activities performed.

The names of bones, muscles, arteries, veins, and nerves are seldom used in the electrology office. However, an understanding, of body structures will help make you more proficient in giving treatments.

THE SKELETAL SYSTEM

The **skeletal system** *(SKEL e tal SIS tem)* is the physical foundation of the body. It is composed of differently shaped bones united by movable and immovable joints.

Bone is the hardest structure of the body other than teeth. It is composed of fibrous tissues firmly bound together, and is about one-third organic and two-thirds inorganic.

The scientific study of bones and their structure and functions is called **osteology** *(os tee OL o jee).* Os is the technical term for bone.

The following are the functions of bone:

1. To give shape and strength to the body.
2. To protect organs from injury.
3. To serve as attachments for muscles.
4. To act as levers for all bodily movements.

THE MUSCULAR SYSTEM

The **muscular** *(MUS kyoo lar)* system covers, shapes, and supports the skeleton. Its function is to produce all movements of the body.

Myology *(meye OL o jee)* is the study of the structure, functions, and diseases of the muscles.

No outward sign of human life is more distinctive than that of muscular movement.

The muscular system consists of over 500 muscles, large and small, comprising 40% to 50% of the weight of the human body.

Muscles are contractile fibrous tissue on which the various movements of the body depend for their variety and action. The muscular system relies upon the skeletal and nervous systems for its activities.

There are three kinds of muscular tissues. They are:

1. Striated (striped) or voluntary, which are controlled by the will, such as those of the face, arms, and legs.
2. Nonstriated (smooth) or involuntary, which function without the action of the will, such as those of the stomach and intestines.
3. Cardiac (heart muscle), which is the heart itself, and is not duplicated anywhere else in the body.

Nucleus

Striated Muscle Cell

Tendon

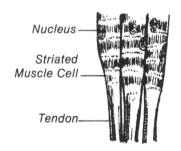

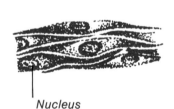

Nucleus

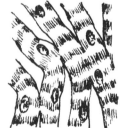

Striated (Striped) Muscle Cells *Nonstriated (Smooth) Muscle Cells* *Cardiac (Heart) Muscle Cells*

Stimulation of Muscles

Muscular tissue may be stimulated by any of the following:

1. Chemicals (certain acids and salts)
2. Massage (hand massage and electric vibrator)
3. Electric current (high-frequency and faradic current)
4. Light rays (infrared rays and ultraviolet rays)
5. Heat rays (heating lamps and heating caps)
6. Moist heat (steamers or moderately warm steam towels)
7. Nerve impulses (through the nervous system)

THE NERVOUS SYSTEM

Neurology *(nuu ROL o jee)* is the branch of science that deals with the nervous system and its disorders.

The **nervous** *(NUR vus)* system is one of the most important systems of the body. It controls and coordinates the functions of all the other systems and makes them work harmoniously.

The main purpose in studying the nervous system is to understand what effects electrology treatments have on the body as a whole, especially as related to pain.

Divisions of the Nervous System

The principal parts that compose the nervous system are the brain, the spinal cord, and their nerves. The nervous system is composed of three main divisions:

1. The **cerebro-spinal** *(se REE broh SPEYE nahl)* or central nervous system.
2. The **peripheral** *(pe RIF er rahl)* nervous system.
3. The **sympathetic** *(sim pah THET ik)* nervous system.

Cerebro-Spinal System

The cerebro-spinal nervous system consists of the brain and spinal cord. The following are its functions:

1. To control consciousness and all mental activities.
2. To control the voluntary functions of the five senses, such as seeing, smelling, tasting, feeling and hearing.
3. To control voluntary muscle actions, such as all body movements and facial expressions.

Peripheral System

The sensory and motor nerve fibers extend from the brain and spinal cord and are distributed to all parts of the body; they are referred to as the peripheral system. Their function is to carry messages to and from the central nervous system.

Sympathetic Nervous System

The sympathetic nervous system is related structurally to the cerebro-spinal (central) nervous system, but functions independently of the will.

The sympathetic nervous system is very important in the operation of the internal body functions, such as breathing, circulation, digestion, and glandular activities. Its main purpose is to regulate these internal operations, keeping them in balance and working properly.

Neurons

A **neuron** *(NOOR on)*, or nerve cell, is the structural unit of the nervous system. It is composed of a cell body and fibers called cell processes. The cell body stores energy and food for the cell processes, which carry the nerve impulses through the body. Most nerve cells are contained in the brain and spinal cord.

Nerves

Nerves are long, white cords made up of fibers that carry messages to and from various parts of the body. Nerves originate in the brain and spinal cord and branch to all parts of the body, furnishing both sensation and motion.

Nerves are nourished through blood vessels and lymphatics.

Nerve Cell

A Neuron

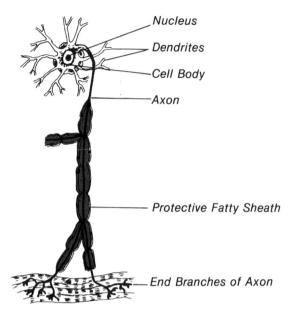

Nucleus

Dendrites

Cell Body

Axon

Protective Fatty Sheath

End Branches of Axon

Types of Nerves   Sensory nerves carry impulses or messages from the sense organs to the brain, where sensations of touch, cold, heat, sight, hearing, taste, smell, and pain are experienced.

Motor nerves carry impulses from the brain to the muscles. The transmitted impulses produce movement.

Sensory nerves are situated near the surface of the skin. Motor nerves are in the muscles. As impulses pass from the sensory nerves to the brain and back over the motor nerves to the muscles, a complete circuit is established and movement of the muscle results.

Nerve Reflex   A nerve reflex is the path traveled by a nerve impulse, through the spinal cord and brain, in response to a stimulus. An example of this is the quick removal of the hand from a hot object. A reflex act does not have to be learned.

Stimulation of the nerves causes muscles to contract and expand. Heat on the skin causes relaxation; cold causes contraction.

Nerve stimulation may be attained by any of the following:

1. Chemicals (certain acids or salts)
2. Electrical current (high-frequency)
3. Light rays (infrared)
4. Heat rays (heating lamps and heating caps)
5. Moist heat (steamers or moderately warm steam towels)

The Brain   The brain is the largest mass of nerve tissue in the body and is contained in the cranium. It is considered to be the central power station of the body, sending and receiving telegraphic messages.

The Spinal Cord

The spinal cord is composed of masses of nerve cells with fibers running upward and downward. It originates in the brain and extends down to the lower part of the trunk. It is enclosed and protected by the spinal column.

Thirty-one pairs of spinal nerves, which extend from the spinal cord, are distributed to the muscles and skin of the trunk and limbs.

Some of the spinal nerves supply the internal organs controlled by the sympathetic nervous system.

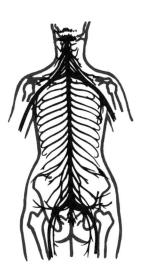

The central nervous system includes the brain and spinal cord. The peripheral nervous system includes the cranial and spinal nerves. The autonomic nervous system controls the smooth muscles of the gastrointestinal tract, the cardio-vascular system and glandular secretions.

THE CIRCULATORY SYSTEM

The **circulatory** *(SUR kyoo la tohr ee)* or **vascular** *(VAS kyoo lar)*, system is vitally important to the maintenance of good health. Proper circulation keeps the hair, skin, and nails healthy looking.

The vascular system controls the circulation of the blood through the body by means of the heart and the blood vessels (the arteries, veins, and capillaries).

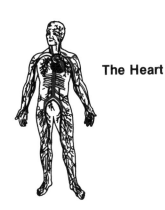

The Heart

The heart is an efficient pump. It keeps the blood moving within the circulatory system.

The heart is a muscular, cone-shaped organ, about the size of a closed fist. It is located in the chest cavity and is enclosed in a membrane, the **pericardium** *(per i CAHR dee um)*. The **vagus** *(VAY gus)* nerve and nerves from the sympathetic nervous system regulate the heartbeat. In a normal adult, the heart beats about 72 to 80 times per minute.

Blood Vessels

The arteries, capillaries and veins are tube-like in construction. They transport blood to and from the heart and to the tissues of the body.

Arteries *(AHR te rees)* are thick-walled muscular and elastic tubes that carry pure blood from the heart to the capillaries.

Capillaries *(KAP i ler ees)* are minute, thin-walled blood vessels that connect the smaller arteries with the veins. Through their walls, the tissues receive nourishment and eliminate waste products.

Cross Section of a Vein

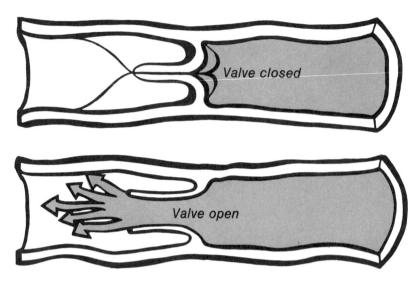

Valve closed

Valve open

Veins are thin-walled blood vessels that are less elastic than arteries. They contain cup-like valves to prevent back-flow, and carry impure blood from the various capillaries back to the heart. The veins are located closer to the outer surface of the body than the arteries.

Blood Circulation

The blood is in constant circulation. There are two systems that take care of this circulation:

1. **Pulmonary** *(PUHL mon air ee)* circulation is the blood circulation that goes from the heart to the lungs to be purified with oxygen, and then returns to the heart.
2. General circulation is the blood circulation from the heart throughout the body and back again to the heart.

The Blood

Blood is the nutritive fluid flowing through the circulatory system. It is a sticky, salty fluid, with a normal temperature that remains at 98.6° F (37° C). It makes up about one-twentieth of the weight of the body. From eight to ten pints of blood fill the blood vessels of an adult.

Blood Cells

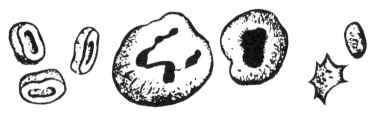

Red Corpuscles   *White Corpuscles*   *Platelets*

Some characteristics of blood are as follows:

Color of blood. The blood is bright red in the arteries (except in the pulmonary artery) and dark red in the veins (except in the pulmonary vein). This change in color is due to the gain of oxygen as the blood passes through the lungs, and the loss of oxygen as it passes through the rest of the body.

Composition of blood. One-third of the blood is composed of red and white corpuscles and blood platelets. The remaining two-thirds is plasma. The function of red corpuscles (red blood cells) is to carry oxygen to the cells. White corpuscles (white blood cells) function by destroying disease-causing germs.

Blood platelets. Blood platelets are much smaller than red blood cells. They play an important part in the clotting of blood over a wound.

Plasma. Plasma is the fluid part of the blood in which the red and white blood cells and platelets flow. It is straw-like in color. About nine-tenths of the plasma is water, and it carries food and secretions to the cells, and carbon dioxide from the cells.

Chief Functions of the Blood

The primary functions of the blood are to:

1. Carry water, oxygen, food, and secretions to all cells of the body.
2. Carry away carbon dioxide and waste products to be eliminated by the lungs, skin, kidneys and large intestine.
3. Help to equalize the body temperature, protecting the body from extreme heat and cold.
4. Aid in protecting the body from harmful bacteria and infections, through the action of the white blood cells.
5. Form clots, closing injured blood vessels and preventing further loss of blood.

The Lymph-Vascular System

The **lymph-vascular** *(limf VAS kyoo lar)* system, also called lymphatic system, is the drainage system for the body tissues. Lymphatic capillaries serve as drains and join and form the larger lymphatic vessels. Cellular products and fluid pass into the lymphatic capillaries and are then called lymph. Before lymph reaches the veins, it is filtered through nodes and then returned to the blood. The lymph carries nourishment from the blood to the cells and removes waste from the cells.

The main function of lymphatic tissue is to remove bacteria and foreign materials, to manufacture lymphocytes which make up some of the white blood cells, and produce antibodies to combat infection. The tonsils are an example of lymphoid tissues.

THE GLANDULAR SYSTEM

Glands are specialized organs which vary in size and function. The blood and nerves are intimately connected with the glands. The nervous system controls the functional activities of the glands. The glands have the ability to remove certain constituents from the blood and to convert them into new compounds.

There are two main sets of glands:

1. One group is called the duct glands, because they possess canals (called ducts) which lead from the gland to a particular part of the body. The sweat and oil glands of the skin, as well as intestinal glands, belong to this group.
2. The other group, known as ductless glands, comprises the endocrine system. These glands produce hormones which are secreted into the bloodstream. The endocrine system influences hair growth and is often the cause of excess hair. You will find detailed information on the endocrine system in Chapter 12.

THE EXCRETORY SYSTEM

The **excretory** *(EK skre tohr ee)* system, including the kidneys, liver, skin, intestines, and lungs, purifies the body by eliminating waste matter.

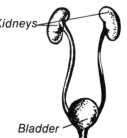

The kidneys excrete urine.
The liver discharges bile pigments.
The skin eliminates perspiration.
The large intestine evacuates decomposed and undigested food.
The lungs exhale carbon dioxide

The metabolism of the cells of the body forms various toxic substances which, if retained, would poison the body.

THE RESPIRATORY SYSTEM

The **respiratory** *(RES pi rah tohr ee)* system is situated in the chest cavity and is protected by the ribs. The **diaphragm** *(DEYE ah fram)*, a muscular partition which controls breathing, separates the chest from the **abdominal** *(ab DOM i nahl)* regions.

The lungs are spongy tissues composed of microscopic cells into which the inhaled air penetrates. These tiny air cells are enclosed in a skin-like tissue. Behind this, the fine capillaries of the blood vascular system are found.

Oxygen is more essential than either food or water. Although a man or woman may live more than sixty days without food, and a few days without water, if air is excluded for even a few minutes, death results.

DIGESTIVE SYSTEM

The **digestive** *(deye JES tiv)* system changes food into **soluble** *(SOL yoo bul)* form, suitable for the body's cells to use. Digestion is started in the mouth and completed in the small **intestine** *(in TES tin)*. From the mouth, the food passes down the **pharynx** *(FAR ingks)* and the **esophagus** *(i SOF a gus)*, or food pipe, and into the stomach. The food is completely digested in the small intestine. The large intestine (colon) absorbs water and stores the refuse for elimination through the rectum. The complete digestion of food takes about nine hours.

Digestion is the process of converting food into a form which can be assimilated by the body. Responsible for the chemical changes in food are the **enzymes** *(EN zeyems)* present in the digestive secretions. Digestive enzymes are chemicals which change certain kinds of food into a form capable of being used by the body.

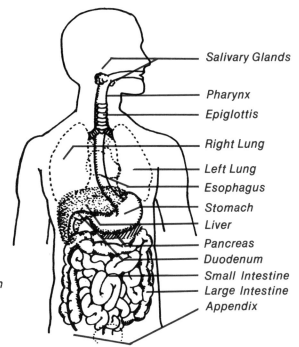

Salivary Glands

Pharynx
Epiglottis

Right Lung

Left Lung
Esophagus
Stomach
Liver
Pancreas
Duodenum
Small Intestine
Large Intestine
Appendix

Diagram illustrating the Human Alimentary Canal with its Principal Digestive Glands.

Digestion and the Skin

The correct functioning of the digestive system is important to the appearance of the skin. The skin is nourished by the bloodstream, and a well-balanced diet supplies the nutrients needed to keep the skin healthy and attractive. The body also needs a sufficient amount of fluids and water to keep the skin from dehydrating.

Fatigue, poor habits of elimination, and intense emotions such as excitement, anger, and stress, can seriously disturb digestion and lead to skin and possibly hair growth problems. Relaxation, peace of mind, and a general sense of well-being are beneficial to the client during electrology treatment.

QUESTIONS FOR REVIEW

1. What are the functions of the bones?
2. What are the three kinds of muscular tissue and where is each muscle type found?
3. What are the divisions of the nervous system? What is the function of each division?
4. What are the two systems of blood circulation and how do they work?
5. What are the functions of glands?
6. What is the importance of the excretory system?
7. What is the composition of the lungs?
8. What is the function of the digestive system?

Chapter 12 The Endocrine System

LEARNING OBJECTIVES

Successful mastery of the material in this chapter will be indicated when you can:

1. List the glands and explain which ones can cause excess hair growth.
2. Explain how the placenta can perform an endocrine function and how this can cause excess hair to grow.

INTRODUCTION

The **endocrine system** is a major body system important to the electrologist. The endocrine system is composed of ductless glands whose function is to secrete chemical substances, known as hormones, directly into the bloodstream. Hormones are responsible for various body functions. Hormonal disturbances are often linked to growth of excess hair.

The Endocrine System

(Both male and female glands are shown.)

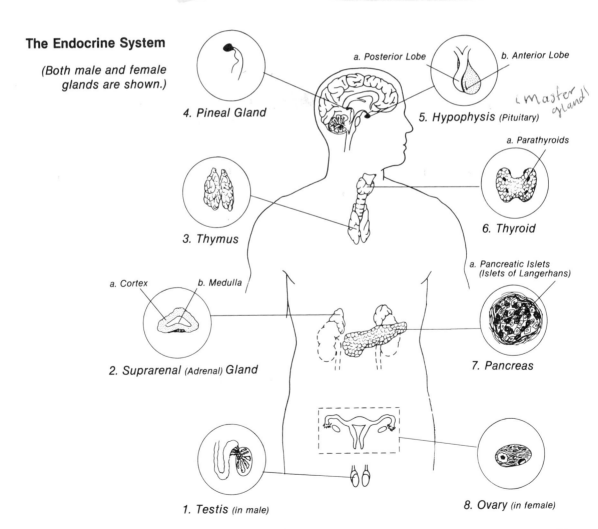

4. Pineal Gland

a. Posterior Lobe   b. Anterior Lobe

5. Hypophysis *(Pituitary)*   *(master gland)*

a. Parathyroids

6. Thyroid

3. Thymus

a. Pancreatic Islets (Islets of Langerhans)

a. Cortex   b. Medulla

2. Suprarenal *(Adrenal)* Gland

7. Pancreas

1. Testis *(in male)*

8. Ovary *(in female)*

THE GLANDS   We will now briefly study those endocrine glands which affect hair growth on the body.

Pituitary Gland   The **pituitary gland** *(pi TOO i ter ee)* is located at the base of the brain and is connected to it. The pituitary gland is composed of three sections known as the **anterior, intermediate,** and **posterior** lobes. These lobes can almost be considered three different glands as each secretes different hormones.

(master gland)

Excess production of hormones from the pituitary can result in superfluous hair.

1. **Anterior lobe** *(an TEER i or lohb).* This portion of the pituitary regulates the growth hormone. An excess of this hormone will cause enlarged hands, feet, and faces, and excess hair. The regulating hormone for the adrenal cortex is also secreted here, and again, an oversecretion will cause hirsutism. Lastly, the anterior lobe secretes the hormone that activates the thyroid gland.
2. **Intermediate lobe** *(in tur MEE di it).* The intermediate lobe secretes a hormone which stimulates pigment.
3. **Posterior lobe** *(po STEER i or).* The posterior lobe produces two component hormones which assist in childbearing and prevent water loss from the kidneys. Stress can cause overproduction and excessive hair growth.

Thyroid Gland   The **thyroid gland** *(THEYE roid)* is composed of two lobes located on either side of the windpipe. The thyroid secretes two hormones which regulate metabolism. Specialists are now beginning to believe that excessive production of these thyroid hormones can cause excess hair.

Adrenal Glands   The two **adrenal glands** *(a DREE nahl)* are located above the kidneys. The outer portion of the adrenal gland secretes a hormone which regulates the metabolism of fats, proteins, and carbohydrates. The outer portion also produces sex hormones. Women can suffer from hirsutism when these hormones are excreted in excess.

The inner portion of the adrenal gland secretes hormones which regulate the nervous system and increase blood pressure and heart rate.

Pancreas   The **pancreas** *(PAN kree as)* is a compound gland located on the abdominal wall behind the stomach. It secretes the hormone insulin, which regulates the metabolism of carbohydrates. Excess facial hair or beards on women have been linked to malfunctions of the pancreas.

Ovaries   The **ovaries** *(OH va reez)* are the female sex glands. They are located in the pelvic cavity. They produce egg cells, and the hormones **estrogen** *(ES tro jen)* and **progesterone** *(pro JES te rohn).* All secondary sex characteristics are dependent on the secretion of these hormones. Malfunctioning of the ovaries can cause serious hirsutism.

Testes   The **testes** *(TES teez)* are the male sex glands. They are located in the scrotal sac, and produce sperm cells and the hormone **androgen** *(AN dro jen),* which regulates sex characteristics and the reproductive system. An oversecretion of this hormone can cause male hirsutism.

PLACENTA   The **placenta** *(pla SEN ta)* is an organ that develops during pregnancy. It performs an endocrine function by secreting a hormone similar to those secreted by the pituitary gland. Somehow this overabundance stimulates the whole endocrine system and increases blood supply, which can cause excess hair growth in many women. This hair growth is usually not severe.

QUESTIONS FOR REVIEW:
1. What are the glands that can cause excess hair growth?
2. How does the placenta perform an endocrine function? How can this cause excess hair to grow?

Chapter 13 Excess Hair, Hirsutism, and Hypertrichosis

LEARNING OBJECTIVES
Successful mastery of the material in this chapter will be indicated when you can:

1. Give the three categories of electrology treatment.
2. Define and state the cause of hirsutism.
3. Explain the difference between hypertrichosis and hirsutism.
4. Describe how hormonal changes can cause excess hair.
5. List examples of iatrogenic hirsutism.
6. State what glands can cause excess hair.
7. List six other causes of excess hair.

INTRODUCTION
The human body is covered with hair follicles. Hair follicles may be dormant, growing no hair; or they may grow fine, vellus hair or thick, terminal hair.

The distribution of hair varies according to race. Negroids, Orientals, Mongolians, and American Indians have less hair then Caucasians. Caucasians of Mediterranean origin are more hirsute than Nordic or other light-skinned Caucasians.

Excess hair has been an esthetic problem for women for thousands of years. Excess hair, from the point of view of a female patient, is usually hair on the upper lip, chest, breast, abdomen, and on the back. The amount of hair considered unattractive and excessive is relative to the region of the world and the time in history.

Hirsute *(HUR soot)* men are disturbed by excessive hair growth on the bridge of the nose, top of the nose, ears, cheekbone area, neck, back, chest, arms, and hands. Some men may have unusual amounts of hair even on their legs.

CATEGORIES OF ELECTROLOGY TREATMENT
Electrology treatment is divided into three categories. The first is **cosmetic correction.** This type of treatment is strictly for cosmetic effect and the hair treated is not considered abnormal hair growth. Treatment of the hairline, eyebrows, underarms, and sometimes the legs and arms, as well as fine, vellus hair that can hardly be seen, fall into this category.

The second category is **psychological cosmetic corrective treatment.** This type of treatment attempts to relieve the anguish that a patient develops due to the perceived disfigurement of a hirsute condition.

The third category is **surgical correction.** This includes the delicate treatment of eyelashes, ingrown lashes, and the removal of ingrown hairs where the skin must be broken first.

The electrologist must inquire about state regulations and insurance concerning surgical correction. This type of treatment should only be given after medical consultation, and if it is permissible in your state.

In order to achieve successful treatment, it is important that the practitioner understand both the biological and the psychological aspects of the patient's problem.

HIRSUTISM

Hirsutism *(HUR soot izm)* is a term usually reserved for females. It refers to the growth of hair on the face and body which is usually characteristic of masculinity. Hirsutism is caused by an overabundance of the hormone androgen in the blood. The dormant follicles are stimulated to grow hair, and existing vellus and **terminal hairs grow larger in diameter.**

HYPERTRICHOSIS

When the excess hair is confined to areas of the arms, legs, feet, and sometimes, the neck and back, it is called **hypertrichosis** *(HEYE per treye KOH sis).* It is not characterized as masculine. The vellus and terminal hair increases in quantity but **not necessarily in diameter.** Both men and women may be characterized as having hypertrichosis.

All hair growth, normal or abnormal, is regulated by hormones. It is the oversecretion of male hormones that causes excessive hair growth. Research has established that most excess hair is due to a combination of overabundant **androgen** *(AN dro jen)* and an enzyme in the follicle that is sensitive to androgen increase.

HORMONAL CAUSES OF EXCESS HAIR
Heredity and Puberty

As a person becomes an adult, secondary sex traits appear. For the female, breasts develop, menstruation begins, and pubic and **axillary** *(AK sil er ee)*, or armpit hair, appears. For the male, a beard, axillary and pubic hair, and a deepening of the voice occur. The adjustment of hormone levels at this time can result in excess hair and acne.

Age

As a woman ages, her reproductive organs change. She enters menopause and her female hormone, **estrogen** *(ES tro jen)* level decreases substantially. This results in an increase of the male hormones, **testosterone** *(tes TOS te rohn)* and androgen, which can cause excessive hair to begin to grow.

Many males also begin to grow excess hair in mid-life, especially on the back and ears.

Pregnancy

It is not uncommon for a woman to lose hair on her head during pregnancy and, at the same time, to develop **superfluous** *(soo PUR floo us)* hair on the face and chest. After pregnancy, the hair on the head will usually regrow, but the superfluous hair rarely disappears. *more than required*
excessive hair

IATROGENIC HIRSUTISM

Iatrogenic *(eye ah tro JEN ik)* hirsutism refers to superfluous hair growth caused by drugs. Let us examine the most common types of drugs that can cause excessive hair to grow. Most of these drugs are derived from hormones.

Many patients claim that they begin to grow excess hair when they begin taking birth control pills. Strangely enough, the same oral contraceptive may also be prescribed by a physician when a patient with an irregular menstrual cycle is experiencing hair growth.

There are many other types of medications that can cause excessive hair growth. Treatment for discomfort during menopause, for seizures, and for various types of **gynecological** *(geye ne ko LOJ i kahl)* illnesses can all cause increased hair growth. Drugs used to treat high blood pressure, kidney disease, and low blood sugar have also been recorded as stimulating excessive hair growth. **Chemotherapy** *(kee moh THER a pee)* can cause excessive hair growth on the faces of female cancer patients, and antibiotics used to treat tuberculosis can cause excessive hair growth in children.

GLANDULAR CAUSES OF EXCESS HAIR

The following causes of excess hair are directly related to a particular gland of the endocrine system. (The endocrine system is discussed in detail in Chapter 12.)

Ovaries

The **Stein Leventhal** *(steyen LEV en thaul)* Syndrome occurs when the ovaries have more than one cyst, stimulating high levels of androgen. The patient is usually overweight, has irregular menstrual cycles, is generally infertile, and is sometimes masculine in appearance. Because of overproduction of androgens, the patient develops hirsutism. The face and most of the body can become very hirsute.

Patients with this condition may need many years of electrology treatment. Until the cause is treated medically, dormant follicles will continue to be stimulated, causing even more hair growth.

A **tumor of the ovary** can cause patients to develop hirsutism and take on masculine characteristics. This development of male secondary characteristics in a woman increases muscles, broadens shoulders, and enlarges the clitoris. Acne often develops and the voice deepens. These tumors, as well as cysts, can be removed surgically, and the syndrome is usually corrected. The hirsutism rarely disppears after medical treatment, however, and must be treated by electrology, although more hair seldom grows.

Pituitary Gland

master gland

Acromegaly *(AK roh MEG ah lee)* is the result of oversecretion of the growth hormone from the pituitary. When the pituitary gland secretes too much hormone due to stimulation by a tumor, enlargement of the hands, feet, face, and other parts of the body will result.

The pituitary hormone also directly stimulates the adrenal glands, causing excessive secretion of androgen. Both men and women can suffer from acromegaly and become hirsute.

Cushing Syndrome

Cushing Syndrome is a result of a pituitary tumor. Such tumors cause excess amounts of **glucocorticoids** *(gloo ko KOR ti koids)* or excess adrenocorticotrophic hormone *(ad REE noh KOHR tee koh TROF ik)* more commonly known as **ACTH**. These increases lead to higher levels of androgen and adrenal hormones.

The adult female will develop a moon face. Fat will develop on the neck and trunk of the body while the arms and legs will be normal or thin by comparison. Again, the increased androgen levels will cause severe hirsutism.

Adrenal Gland

The **Archard-Theirs** Syndrome is also known as "the diabetes of bearded women." A patient with this disease is usually obese, hirsute, and has diabetes, hypertension, and excess levels of androgen hormones. Achard-Theirs can be distinguished from the Cushing Syndrome. The arms and legs are also obese, and the face is not moon-shaped.

The term **adrenal hyperplasia** *(a DREE nal HEYE per PLAZ ee ah)* simply means an excessive growth of normal cells in the adrenal gland. The enlargement of the gland that results increases androgen hormone production. When this occurs in a young female before puberty, male characteristics and hirsutism will result.

Women can also develop this syndrome in their thirties or forties. At this time they will usually develop excess hair and acne. Fortunately, these problems are rare.

The electrologist must never diagnose disease or prescribe medication.

Awareness of the symptoms of these syndromes will help you be more sensitive to your patient's needs. If you note these symptoms, or if your patient has an irregular menstrual cycle (or none at all), you should suggest she see a gynecologist, endocrinologist, or her physician. You can then treat the resulting excess hair while the physician treats the medical cause.

Physicians may also prescribe hormone medication to treat these or other syndromes. *You should never tell patients to stop the medication.* It is advisable, though, to inform them that it may be causing the excess hair, especially if the growth began after medication started.

OTHER CAUSES OF EXCESS HAIR

Hysterectomies

Hysterectomies *(his teh REK to mees)*, the removal of the female reproductive organs, may cause severe stress, especially to younger patients who desire a family. When the ovaries are removed, no estrogen is secreted. The testosterone and androgen levels are then proportionally higher, stimulating dormant hair follicles to grow hair.

Stress

It is very common for electrologists to notice excess hair on female patients enduring severe stress or trauma. The adrenal gland secretes larger amounts of androgen at such times. Many women in stress-related businesses are beginning to notice superfluous hair on their faces. Women who are institutionalized for psychological problems are usually under great stress and often exhibit excessive hair growth.

Atavistic Syndrome   Sometimes young girls will exhibit hypertrichosis before puberty. The hair grows along the spine, back, arms and sometimes the underarms. This is called the **atavistic** *(at ah VIS tik SIN drohm)* **syndrome.** The cause of this condition is not yet known. The theory is that the hypertrichosis is due to heredity.

With the parents' permission, these young children can be treated successfully.

Topical Causes   Topical causes of excess hair stimulate the blood supply to the hair follicle. The most common irritants are the sun, x rays, ultraviolet light, and some scar-causing injuries. Excess hair growth from topical causes is usually not severe.

Obesity   Many of the causes of hypertrichosis and hirsutism are related to **obesity** *(oh BEE si tee)*. Not all cases of obesity are disease-related. It is common, however, for obese women to develop hirsutism. Scientific studies have shown that these individuals develop a synthetic hormone that causes stimulation of the follicles.

Anorexia Nervosa   **Anorexia Nervosa** *(an o REK see ah nur VOH sah)* is a disorder characterized by voluntary starvation. This disorder can result in hirsute characteristics. Anorexic patients can be treated successfully, although a physician should first be consulted.

QUESTIONS FOR REVIEW
1. What are the three categories of electrology treatment?
2. What is hirsutism and what causes it?
3. What is the difference between hypertrichosis and hirsutism?
4. How can hormonal changes cause excess hair?
5. What are examples of iatrogenic hirsutism?
6. What glands can cause excess hair?
7. What are six other causes of excess hair?

Chapter 14 Physiology and Histology of the Skin

LEARNING OBJECTIVES   Successful mastery of the material in this chapter will be indicated when you can:

1. Describe the two forms of keratin.
2. List the appendages of the skin and identify their parts.
3. Describe the layers of the epidermis, dermis, and subcutaneous tissue.
4. List the classifications of nerves and explain their functions.
5. Explain the sources of coloring and elasticity in the skin.
6. Describe the functions and structures of the glands of the skin.
7. List the functions of the skin.

INTRODUCTION   The scientific study of the skin is of particular importance to the electrologist. The skin is the largest organ of the body and performs many vital functions required for health and beauty. Healthy skin is moist, soft, flexible, slightly acidic, and is free from blemishes and disease. The skin's texture should be smooth and fine-grained.

The skin varies in thickness from one-twelfth to one-fifth of an inch (.212 cm to .508 cm). The skin is thinnest on the eyelids and thickest on the palms of the hands and the soles of the feet.

Every inch of skin contains millions of cells and a network of nerves and blood vessels. In addition, the skin contains pores that are the openings for **hair follicles** *(FOL i kels)*, **sebaceous** *(si BAY shus)* **glands,** and sweat glands. The sebaceous glands produce the sebum (oil) that lubricates the skin.

The **epidermis** *(epi DUR mis)* of the skin protects the delicate tissue of the body from injury. This protective ability of the skin is due to the fact that it is made of a substance called keratin.

KERATIN COMPOSITION

Keratin *(KER a tin)* comes in two forms: hard, as in the hair; or soft, as in the skin. Being a protein, it contains substantial amounts of the following elements: carbon, nitrogen, hydrogen, phosphorus, oxygen and sulphur.

Soft Keratin—Soft keratin contains about 2% sulphur, 50% to 75% moisture, and a small percentage of fats. Soft keratin is found in the skin, especially in the layer of the epidermis, where it occurs in the form of flattened cells or as dry scales.

Hard Keratin—Hard keratin, found in hair, has a sulphur content of 4% to 8%, a lower moisture and fat content, and is a particularly tough, elastic material. It forms continuous sheets (fingernails) or long fibers (hair). Hard keratin does not shed, but remains a continuous structure as long as it is in the growing phase.

APPENDAGES OF THE SKIN

Hair Follicle

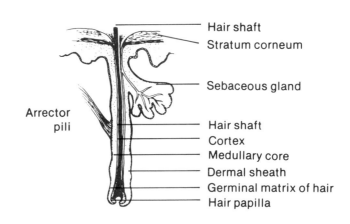

Hair shaft
Stratum corneum

Sebaceous gland

Arrector pili

Hair shaft
Cortex
Medullary core
Dermal sheath
Germinal matrix of hair
Hair papilla

Sebaceous Gland

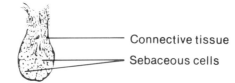

Connective tissue
Sebaceous cells

Sweat Gland

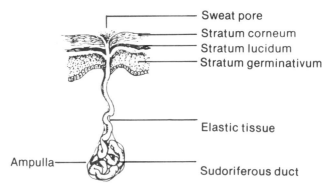

Sweat pore
Stratum corneum
Stratum lucidum
Stratum germinativum

Elastic tissue

Ampulla

Sudoriferous duct

STRUCTURE OF THE SKIN

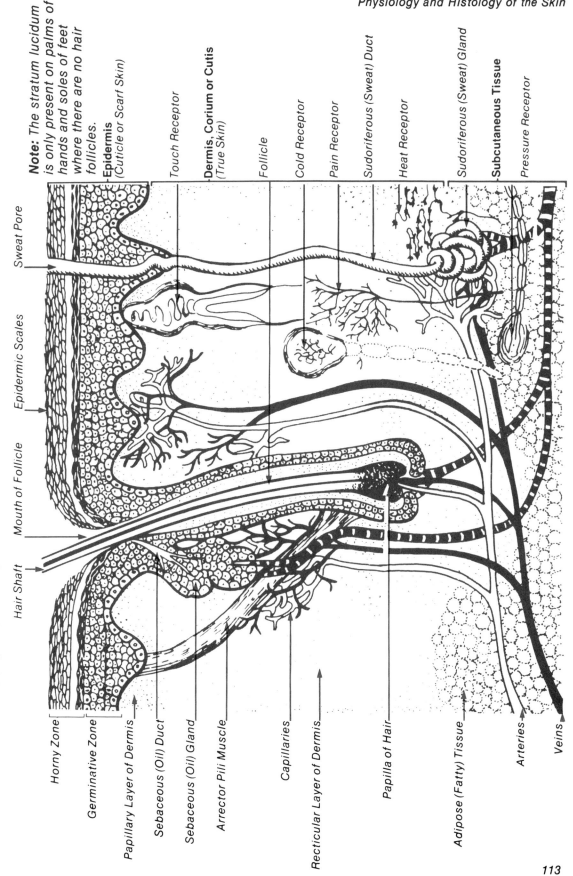

Note: The stratum lucidum is only present on palms of hands and soles of feet where there are no hair follicles.

Epidermis
(Cuticle or Scarf Skin)

Touch Receptor

Dermis, Corium or Cutis
(True Skin)

Follicle

Cold Receptor

Pain Receptor

Sudoriferous (Sweat) Duct

Heat Receptor

Sudoriferous (Sweat) Gland

Subcutaneous Tissue

Pressure Receptor

Sweat Pore

Epidermic Scales

Mouth of Follicle

Hair Shaft

Horny Zone

Germinative Zone

Papillary Layer of Dermis

Sebaceous (Oil) Duct

Sebaceous (Oil) Gland

Arrector Pili Muscle

Capillaries

Recticular Layer of Dermis

Papilla of Hair

Adipose (Fatty) Tissue

Arteries

Veins

113

**STRUCTURES
IN THE SKIN**

**1 Square Inch
Of Skin Contains
(6.452 Sq. Cm)**

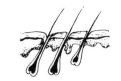

65 hairs

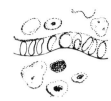

9,500,000 cells

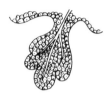

95-100 sebaceous glands

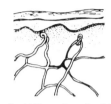

19 yards (17 meters) of blood
vessels

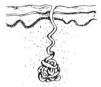

650 sweat glands

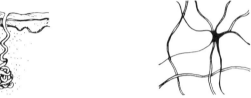

78 yards (70 meters) of nerves

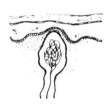

78 sensory apparatuses
for heat

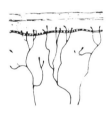

19,500 sensory cells at the
ends of nerve fibers

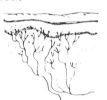

1,300 nerve endings to
record pain

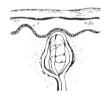

160-165 pressure apparatuses
for the perception of tactile
stimuli

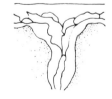

13 sensory apparatuses
for cold

HISTOLOGY OF THE SKIN

The skin contains two clearly defined divisions: the **epidermis** and the **dermis** *(DUR mis)*.

Epidermis

The **epidermis** is the outermost layer of the skin, also known as cuticle or scarf skin. The epidermis forms the protective covering of the skin. It contains no blood vessels, but has many small nerve endings. The epidermis contains the following layers:

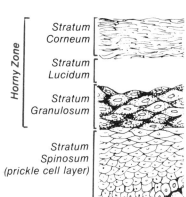

Horny Zone

Stratum Corneum

Stratum Lucidum

Stratum Granulosum

Stratum Spinosum (prickle cell layer)

Germinativum rminative layer or basal layer)

Papillary Layer of Dermis

1. The **stratum corneum** *(STRA tum KOR nee um)*, or horny layer, consists of tightly packed, scale-like cells which are continually being shed and replaced.

2. The **stratum lucidum** *(LOO si dum)*, or clear layer, consists of small, transparent cells through which light can pass.

3. The **stratum granulosum** *(gran yoo LOH sum)*, or glandular layer, consists of cells which look like distinct granules. These cells are almost dead and undergo a change into a horny substance.

4. The **stratum spinosum** *(spi NOH sum)*, or prickle cell layer, is often classified with the stratum germinativum to form the basal layer. Spiny threads join the cells.

5. The **stratum germinativum** *(jer mi nah TIV um)*, formerly known as the stratum mucosum *(myoo KOH sum)*, is composed of several layers of differently shaped cells. The deepest layer is responsible for the growth of the epidermis. It also contains a dark pigment called melanin *(MEL ah nin)*, which protects the sensitive cells from the destructive effects of ultraviolet rays.

NOTE: *Stratum germinativum is also referred to as the* **basal** *(BAYS al)* *or* **Malpighian** *(mal PIG i an) layer.*

The Dermis

The **dermis** is the inner layer of the skin. It may also be called the derma, corium, cutis, or true skin.

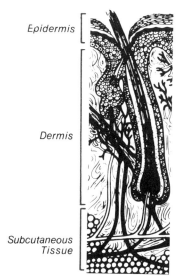

Epidermis

Dermis

Subcutaneous Tissue

The dermis is very sensitive. Within its structure are found numerous blood and lymph vessels, nerves, sweat and oil glands, hair follicles, **arrector pili** *(ah REK tor PI lee) muscles, and papillae. The dermis consists of two layers, the papillary layer, and the reticular layer.*

1. The **papillary** *(PAP i ler ee)* layer lies directly beneath the epidermis. It contains small cone-shaped projections of elastic tissue, called **papillae** *(pa PIL ee)*, that point upward into the epidermis. Some of these papillae contain looped capillaries, while others contain nerve fiber endings called **tactile corpuscles** *(TAK til KOR puh sels)*.

2. The **reticular** *(re TIK yoo lar)* layer contains the following structures:

a. Fat cells
b. Blood vessels
c. Lymph vessels
d. Oil glands

e. Sweat glands
f. Hair follicles
g. Arrector pili muscles

Subcutaneous Tissue

Subcutaneous *(sub kyoo TAY nee us)* tissue is a fatty layer found below the dermis. This tissue, also called adipose, varies in thickness according to the age, sex, and general health of the individual. The subcutaneous layer gives smoothness and contour to the body, contains fat for use as energy, and acts as a protective cushion. Circulation in this area is maintained by a network of blood and lymph vessels.

NOTE: *Some histologists regard the subcutaneous tissue as a continuation of the dermis.*

How the Skin is Nourished

Blood and lymph nourish the skin. From one-half to two-thirds of the total blood supply of the body is distributed to the skin. Essential materials for growth, nourishment, and repair of the skin, hair, and nails are supplied by the blood and lymph. The subcutaneous tissue has networks of arteries and lymphatic vessels, which send their smaller branches to hair papillae, hair follicles, and skin glands. There are numerous capillaries in the skin.

NERVES OF THE SKIN

The skin contains the surface endings of nerve fibers classified as:

1. **Motor nerve fibers,** which are distributed to the arrector pili muscles attached to hair follicles.
2. **Sensory nerve fibers,** which react to heat, cold, touch, pressure and pain.
3. **Secretory nerve fibers,** which are distributed to the sweat and oil glands of the skin.

SENSORY NERVES OF THE SKIN

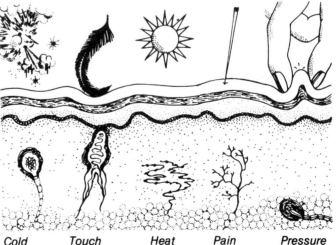

| Cold Receptor | Touch Receptor | Heat Receptor | Pain Receptor | Pressure Receptor |

Sense of Touch   The papillary layer of the dermis provides the sense of touch. Nerves supplying the skin register basic types of sensations: touch, pain, heat, cold, and pressure or deep touch. Nerve endings are most abundant in the fingertips. "Complex sensations," such as the feeling of vibration, seem to depend on a combination of these nerve endings.

COLOR AND ELASTICITY   The color of the skin, whether fair or dark depends primarily on melanin, the coloring matter that is deposited in the stratum germinativum. It also depends to a limited extent on the blood supply to the skin.

The pliability *(pleye ah BIL i tee)* of the skin depends on the elasticity *(ee las TIS i tee)* of the fibers in the dermis. When a person begins to age, the skin begins to lose its elasticity. Small lines begin to form, especially around the eyes and mouth. Factors that can speed aging include: sun, heredity, health, climate, environment, smoking, and diet.

GLANDS OF THE SKIN   The main function of sebum is to act as a shield to prevent moisture from evaporating from the surface of the skin. Sweat keeps the skin naturally moist, preventing dryness.

The skin contains two types of duct glands:

1. The **sudoriferous,** *(SOO do RIF er us)* or sweat glands, excrete sweat.
2. The **sebaceous,** *(si BAY shus)* or oil glands, secrete sebum.

PROTECTIVE ACTION OF SEBUM

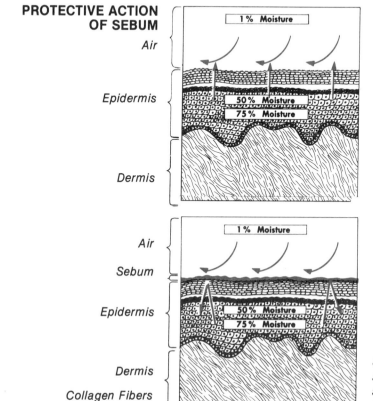

The main function of sebum is to act as a shield that prevents moisture from evaporating from the surface of the skin.

Summer increases the rate of sweating, and this enables the skin to be kept naturally moist, preventing drying and chafing.

Sweat Glands   The sweat glands consist of a coiled base, or **fundus** *(FUN dus)* and a tube-like duct which terminates at the skin surface forming the sweat pore. Practically all parts of the body are supplied with sweat glands, which are more numerous on the palms, soles, forehead, and armpits. The sweat glands regulate body temperature and help to eliminate waste products from the body. Their activity is increased by heat, exercise, emotions, and certain drugs. The excretion of sweat is under the control of the nervous system. Normally, one or two pints of liquids containing salts are eliminated daily through the sweat pores of the skin.

Sweat and Oil Glands

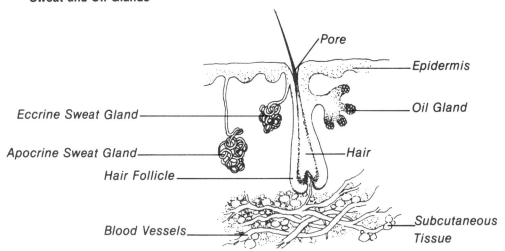

Oil Glands   The oil glands consist of little sacs whose ducts open into the hair follicle. They secrete the sebum *(SEE bum)* which lubricates the skin and helps prevent evaporation of moisture. The palms and soles do not have oil glands. They are found in all other parts of the body, particularly the face.

Sebum is an oily, semifluid substance. Ordinarily it flows through the oil ducts leading into the hair follicles. When the follicle is blocked so that the sebum hardens, however, a blackhead is formed. Deep cleansing of the follicle is of prime importance in keeping the skin free of blemishes.

Water   Another consideration is the effect of water on the skin. The skin, which contains 50% to 75% moisture, is able to maintain this level only by the secretion of sebum which coats its surface. This layer of oil slows down the evaporation of water in the skin and prevents excess moisture from penetrating it. If the natural oils are removed by any means, this protection is lost. Moisture content is vital for electrolysis treatment.

FUNCTIONS OF THE SKIN

The principal functions of the skin are: protection, sensation, heat regulation, excretion, secretion, and absorption.

Protection

The skin protects the body from injury and bacterial invasion. The outermost layer of the epidermis is covered with a thin layer of sebum, which makes it somewhat waterproof. It is also resistant to temperature changes, minor injuries, chemicals, and many microbes. If germs do invade, the skin becomes inflamed and antibodies destroy them.

Sensation

Through its sensory nerve endings, the skin responds to heat, cold, touch, pressure, and pain. A minor burn is very painful, but a deep burn that destroys the nerves may be painless.

Heat Regulation

Heat regulation is a function of the skin, the organ that protects the body from the environment. The healthy body maintains an internal temperature of about 98.6 degrees F (37° C). As changes occur in the outside temperature, the blood vessels and sweat glands of the skin make necessary adjustments. For instance, heat is lost by the evaporation of sweat.

Excretion

Perspiration from the sweat glands is excreted from the skin. Water lost by perspiration carries salt and other chemicals with it.

Secretion

Sebum is secreted by the sebaceous glands. Excessive flow of oil from the oil glands may produce skin problems. Emotional stress many increase the flow of sebum.

Absorption

Absorption *(ab **SORP** shun)* is limited, but does occur. The skin is penetrated by hair follicles with their sebaceous glands and by the pores of the sudoriferous glands. These pockets will allow entry of certain drugs and chemicals into the body. These chemicals may be absorbed to combat infection of the skin (e.g., antiseptic creams and ointments) or they may be used as skin conditioners to help overcome dryness or damage (e.g., vitamin and moisturizing creams).

QUESTIONS FOR REVIEW

1. What are the two forms of keratin?
2. What are the appendages of the skin? Can you identify their parts?
3. What are the layers of the epidermis? The dermis? The subcutaneous tissue?
4. What are the classifications of nerves and what are their functions?
5. What are the sources of coloring and elasticity in the skin?
6. What are the functions and the structures of the glands of the skin?
7. What are the functions of the skin?

Chapter 15 Physiology and Histology of the Hair

LEARNING OBJECTIVES

Successful mastery of the material in this chapter will be indicated when you can:

1. Explain the functions of the hair.
2. List the structures related to the hair.
3. Diagram the structure of an individual hair.
4. Describe the types of hair and their locations.
5. Explain the growth cycles of the hair.
6. Describe the characteristics of the hair.

INTRODUCTION

As a student studying the science of electrology you must understand the hair and its related structures. Knowledge of the functions, structures, and characteristics of the hair will help you ensure quality treatment for your patients.

FUNCTIONS OF HAIR

There are three main functions of the hair. They are **adornment, protection,** and **warmth.**

Adornment

Hair plays a large part in the appearance of an individual. The hairstyle a person chooses reflects their personality, and also often reflects their chosen profession. Some groups of people and some religions have distinctive styles of wearing their hair which identifies them as members of that religion or group. Some primitive societies use the hair to show rank or to indicate ceremony. The American Indians, for example, are well known for distinctive ways of wearing the hair, and the Australian aborigines wail and tear their hair when a member of the tribe dies. Almost all societies use hair to distinguish males from females.

We must not overlook the psychological benefits of the hair. Good physical appearance includes the hair. As practicing electrologists we must consider this, and we should also consider the psychological damage that can occur when a patient has excess hair. We must also keep in mind that only the patient can judge what is excessive for him or her.

Protection

The most important function of hair is to assist the skin in protecting certain areas of the body. The hair may be regarded as a specialized form of skin whose structure is more effective for the purpose of protection. The following are examples of this protective function:

Brain: Over the ages, man has experienced a gradual reduction in body hair. This not true with scalp hair, however, and the main reason for this is the protective function of scalp hair to the delicate brain tissue.

Eyes: The hair of both the eyelashes and the eyebrows performs a protective function for the eye. The eyebrows divert water, perspiration, oils, chemicals, and other solutions. The tissue surrounding the eyes is extremely sensitive. Reflexes cause a shutting of the eyelids so that the lashes can prevent foreign objects from entering the eyes.

Ears and Nose: Special hairs line the delicate passages of the ears and nose. They trap dust, and also serve as a line of defense against bacteria entering the body.

Body: Body hair is present at those joints where muscular action causes friction, such as the armpits. This hair serves as a cushion, and also assists in the evaporation of perspiration from the area.

Warmth

Prehistoric man had a great deal of body hair that certainly insulated him from the elements. Much of this hair has been reduced over the ages as man began to use feathers, hides, and now clothing for this purpose. The scalp hair still performs the function of warmth, however, especially for the ears and the back of the neck.

STRUCTURES RELATED TO THE HAIR
Hair Follicle Formation

dormant-
inactive

The growth of hair is caused by the development of small pockets in the skin, which are called **follicles** *(FOL i kels).*

Quite some time before birth, certain changes take place in the epidermis of a fetus. At first, small pits or depressions develop in the outer layers. Finally, these pits develop into mature follicles. Everyone is born with a set amount of hair follicles. **New hair can grow from dormant hair follicles, but new follicles are never formed.**

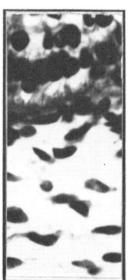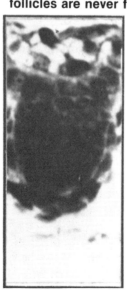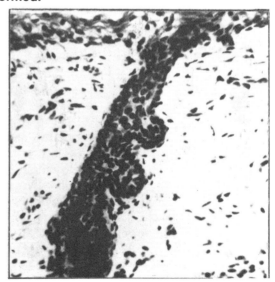

Three stages in the development of hair follicles in the scalp approximately six months before birth. Courtesy: Structure and Function of Skin—Academic Press.

Origin of Follicle and Hair

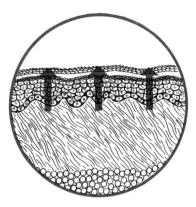

Undeveloped skin

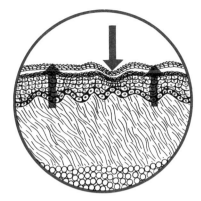

Beginnings of follicle

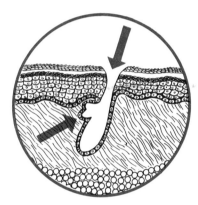

Formation of sebaceous glands

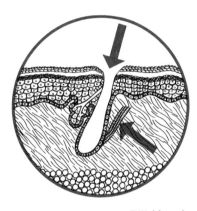

Formation of Arrector Pili Muscle

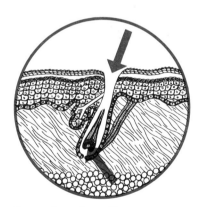

Formation of papilla

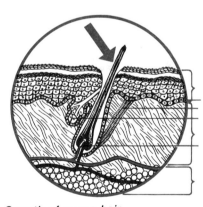

Growth of young hair

EPIDERMIS
Germinal layer
Arrector Pili Muscle
Sebaceous gland
DERMIS
Papilla
SUBCUTANEOUS GLAND

There is no break or hole in the epidermis due to the formation of the follicle. The outside layer of the skin just dips down into the bottom of the follicle and remains as a protective covering.

The epidermis of the follicle, however, does not become dry or scaly. If you were to epilate a hair, you would probably remove a portion of the follicle wall. This is the soft, white tissue at the bottom of the hair shaft called the hair sheath.

Hair Follicle Distribution   Nearly the entire surface of the body is covered with thousands and thousands of these follicles. The palms of the hands, the soles of the feet, the lips, and the eyelids do not contain follicles.

Most follicles on the body remain inactive and never produce hairs. Some follicles only produce hairs at a particular period, such as the development of the beard and pubic hair at puberty. Still others will produce hairs in abnormal situations such as the disturbance of glands and hereditary disorders. This hair growth is of concern to electrologists.

Structure of the Root   There are structures closely associated with the hair root other than the follicle. These include the hair bulb and the hair papilla.

The **hair bulb** is a thickened, club-shaped structure forming the lower part of the hair root. The lower part of the hair bulb is hollowed out to fit over and cover the hair papilla.

The pigment in hair is produced by special cells of the hair bulb. As the hair grows upwards, the pigment is carried into the cortex of the forming hair. Research on hair pigmentation is incomplete, however many experts feel that **lanugo** *(lah **NOO** goh)* hair is lacking a bulb, which would explain its lack of color.

The **papilla** *(pa **PIL** lah)* is a cone-shaped elevation located at the bottom of the hair follicle. It fits into the hair bulb, and is richly supplied with blood and nerves. The papilla is responsible for the growth and regeneration of the hair. It is through the papilla that nourishment reaches the hair bulb.

The other portion of the papilla comes in contact with the germinal matrix and transfers nutrients to the germinative cells. These cells are able to change their supplies of food materials into keratin to form the hair. As long as the papilla functions, the hair will continue to grow. The electrologist needs then, to destroy at least the bottom third of the follicle to ensure that the papilla will not create new cells and produce a new hair.

**Cross Section of the
Hair and Follicle**

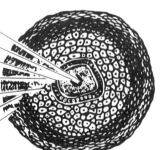

Medulla of hair
Cortex of hair
Cuticle of hair
Inner of epidermic coat
Outer or dermic coat
Inner root sheath
Outer root sheath

**Magnified View
of Hair Cuticle**

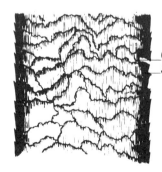

Cuticle
Scales

Cross Section of Hair

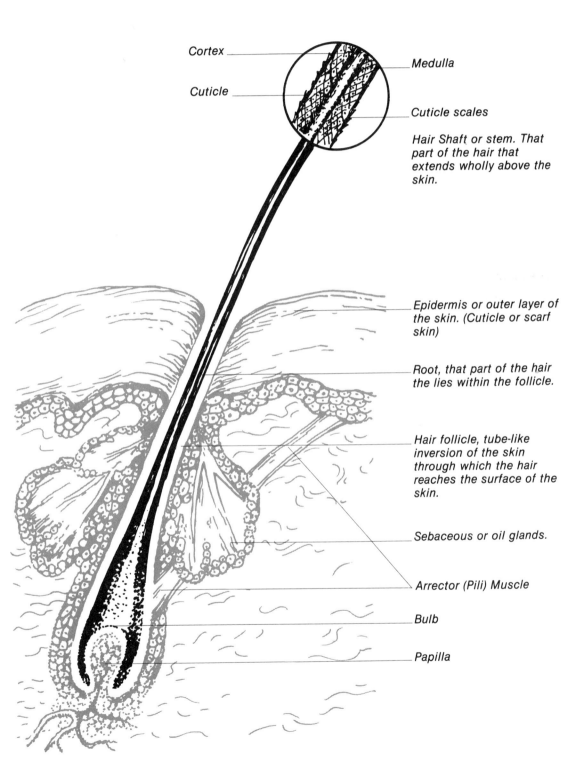

Cortex

Cuticle

Medulla

Cuticle scales

Hair Shaft or stem. That part of the hair that extends wholly above the skin.

Epidermis or outer layer of the skin. (Cuticle or scarf skin)

Root, that part of the hair the lies within the follicle.

Hair follicle, tube-like inversion of the skin through which the hair reaches the surface of the skin.

Sebaceous or oil glands.

Arrector (Pili) Muscle

Bulb

Papilla

Structures Connected to the Hair Follicle

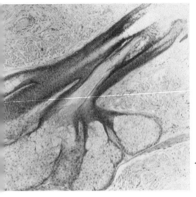

The **arrector pili** *(ah REK tor PI lee)* are small involuntary muscles attached to the underside of a hair follicle. Fear or cold contracts it, causing the hair to stand up straight, causing "gooseflesh." After electrology, gooseflesh will no longer occur because the arrector pili muscles have been destroyed. Eyelash and eyebrow hairs lack arrector pili muscles.

Sebaceous *(si BAY shus)*, or oil glands consist of sac-like structures situated in the dermis. Their ducts are connected to hair follicles. They secrete an oily substance, called **sebum** *(SEE bum)*, which gives luster and pliability to the hair and keeps the skin surface soft and flexible. Much of the activity of this gland is controlled by the endocrine system, and overactivity, especially after puberty, can be an indication of glandular problems. Many of these problems can also be the cause of excess hair.

◄ *Sebaceous glands clustered around a single hair follicle. A special duct or passage ensures a constant flow of natural oils from the skin and hair shaft.*

HAIR STRUCTURE

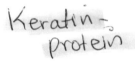

Keratin = protein

The hair is an arrangement of hard **keratin** *(KER ah tin)*. Hair develops by cell reproduction in the germinal layers of the follicle. As the forming hair cells travel up toward the skin surface, they arrange themselves into a specific structure, and gradually harden into a complex fiber.

Three distinct layers with separate functions are formed within the hair fiber. They are:

1. **Cuticle** *(KYOO ti kel)*
2. **Cortex** *(KOR teks)*
3. **Medulla** *(mi DUL ah)*

Magnification of a Cross Section of Hair

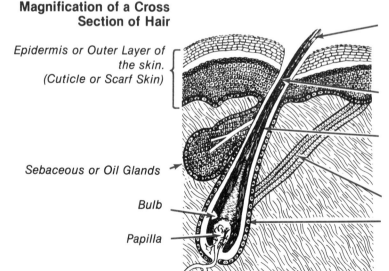

Epidermis or Outer Layer of the skin. (Cuticle or Scarf Skin)

Sebaceous or Oil Glands

Bulb

Papilla

Hair Shaft or Stem, that part of the hair that extends wholly above the skin.

Root, that part of the hair that lies within the follicle.

Hair Follicle, tube-like inversion of the skin through which the hair reaches the surface of the skin.

Arrector Pili Muscle

Germinal Layer

The Cuticle   This is the layer on the outside of the hair shaft. It consists of hard, flattened, horny scales which overlap one another. Five to seven of these layers can be found on the average hair, and up to 16 layers on some hair types.

The cuticle gives the hair its strength and flexibilty. It allows the hair to be bent into shapes, protects the inner layers from the elements, and accounts for the sheen of the hair.

The Cortex   The cortex is the most important layer of the hair and forms 75% to 90% of its bulk or mass. Practically all of the well-known behavior of human hair is due to this important layer.

The physical properties of the hair which depend upon the cortex are:

1. Strength
2. Elasticity
3. Diameter
4. Color
5. Wave

Strength. The nature of the cortex gives the hair great strength. It consists of a complex arrangement of fibrous coils which intertwine. This gives human hair greater strength than a copper wire of the same diameter.

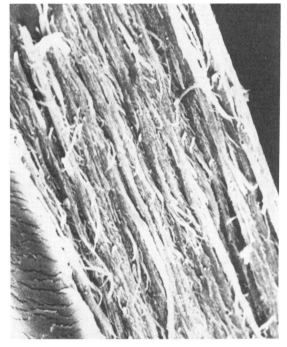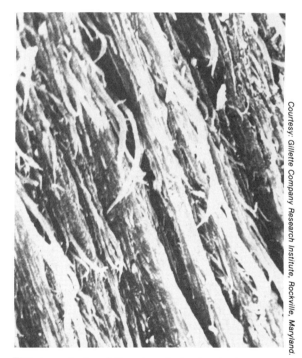

Courtesy: Gillette Company Research Institute, Rockville, Maryland.

Hair fiber with part of the cuticle stripped off exposing the cortex magnified 1470 times. Cortical fibrils can be clearly seen. Notice the vast difference in architecture of the interior of a fiber as compared to the surface.

This is a photo of the same hair structure magnified 4200 times. This gives a closer view of the cortical fibers.

Elasticity. The coil structure of the fibers of the cortex also account for hair's elasticity. The coils are interlocked by hydrogen and salt bonds, which allow the hair to be stretched, and then ensure that it returns to its normal position.

Diameter. The mass of the hair is due to the amount of these fibers in the cortex. The cortex accounts for about 75% to 90% of the hair.

Color. The natural color of the hair is due to melanin granules that are produced at a specialized site on the hair bulb. These granules are released and are trapped in the forming cortex. Lanugo and **vellus** *(VEL us)* hair do not have pigmentation, probably due to incomplete development of the hair root.

Wave. The natural curl pattern of the hair is due to the growth pattern of hair cells in the root. Experts state that genetic factors cause one side of the papilla to produce cells faster, causing uneven growth. The twisting of the fibers into coils (helices) results in a wave pattern. This wave pattern is of importance to the electrologist, as it can distort the follicle, or make the growth pattern difficult to judge.

The Medulla

This is the center of the hair shaft. Its function is unknown, but it probably serves as a channel for nutrients and waste products from the papilla. The medulla has a sponge-like structure, and accounts for a very small portion of the mass of the hair. In all probability, lanugo and vellus hair does not have this layer due to an incomplete or undeveloped hair root.

Magnification of a cross Section of Hair

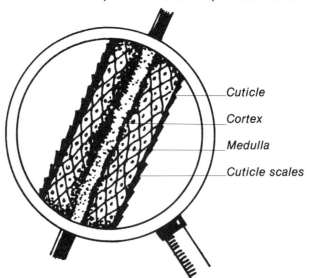

Cuticle

Cortex

Medulla

Cuticle scales

TYPES OF HAIR

There are three main types of hair, each with its own special features. The distinction is usually based on the length of the hair. It does not appear that different types of follicles produce these hairs, but rather that they result from changes in the body or in the papilla. Most of these changes are due to genetic factors, or are a result of hormone imbalances in the body.

Primary Hair

This type of hair is known by several names. Some experts use the terms **vellus** *(VEL us)* and **lanugo** *(lah NOO goh)* interchangeably. Other experts feel there is a distinction between the two. They describe lanugo hair as the fine hair present at birth, and identify vellus hair as the protective fine hair that covers the body later in life. Most of your patients will simply call it "fuzz." There are several distinctive features of primary hair. They are:

1. Lack of medulla.
2. Lack of pigment, which makes the hair difficult to see unless examined in a strong light at the proper angle.
3. Absence of arrector pili muscles, although sebaceous glands **are** present.
4. Short length. Each hair is usually about ½" (1.25 cm).
    The function of primary hair is to aid in the evaporation of perspiration on the body.

Secondary Hair   Secondary hair is the stiff, short, bristly hair of the eyelashes and eyebrows, and can also be found inside the nose and ears, under the arms and in the pubic area.

The follicles of these hairs usually lie at right angles to the surface of the skin, so that the hairs stand straight out away from the skin. They do not possess arrector pili muscles.

The main features of secondary hairs are:

1. A probable increase in thickness and number with age, particularly the eyebrows and edge of ears of an older male.
2. A curved shape, in many cases.
3. A large medulla in many cases.
4. A hair-length range of between ½" and ¾" (1.25 cm and 1.87 cm).
5. More sensitivity to the touch than scalp hairs have, enabling them to act as protection for the eyes, ears, and nose.
6. They are not lost in the normal balding process.

The function of secondary hair is protection. The hair of the eyelashes is controlled by very sensitive reflex actions to prevent foreign objects from entering the eye. The eyebrow hair serves to divert liquids from the eye. The hair of the nose and ears serves as protection against bacteria entering the body. Underarm hair (axillary) and pubic hair fall into this category.

Tertiary Hair   **Tertiary** *(TUR shee er ee)* hair (also kown as terminal hair) is the long, soft, thick hair found on the scalp. It can also be found on the beard and mustache of adult males, and on the legs, arms, and body of both males and females. These hairs grow in groups of two to five, especially on the scalp. In these groups, the hairs may be of different ages and of lengths.

The follicles of these long, soft hairs lie at an angle to the skin. This angle accounts for the growth direction of the hair, and must be considered when inserting the needle during electrology treatment.

Sometimes several follicles merge together to form one opening on the skin surface. This results in multiple hairs or what appears to be several hairs coming from one follicle, a condition that can cause particular problems for the practitioner.

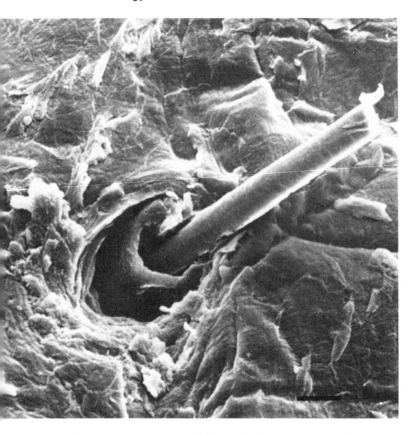

Single hair growing from follicle, magnified 600 times. This is an excellent view of the follicle opening and the sheath around the base of the hair.

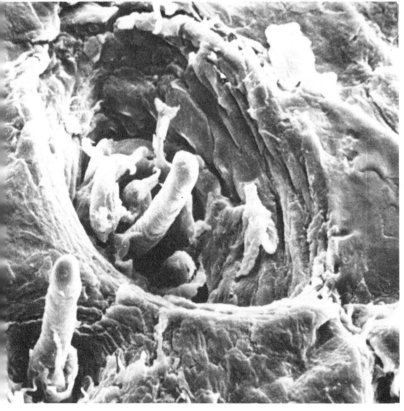

Multiple hairs growing from what appears to be a single follicle, magnified 630 times. Notice follicle architecture which is clearly shown in the center. Courtesy: Gillette Company Research Institute, Rockville, Maryland.

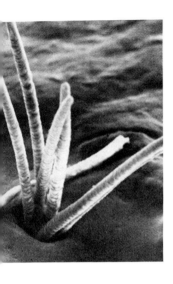

Multiple hairs growing from what appears to be a single follicle, magnified 780 times, obtained from the forehead of a young male. Courtesy: Gillette Company Research Institute, Rockville, Maryland.

Tertiary hair is pigmented. It is only in the case of albinism and aging that tertiary hair is white or gray.

This type of hair often possesses a natural wave. The electrologist will need to cut wavy or curly hair to a short length so as to judge the growth direction of the hair.

Each hair has at least one sebaceous gland associated with the follicle. The function of the gland is to produce a natural oil (sebum). This oil forms a film on the outside of the hair shaft and the outer layer of the epidermis.

Each hair has arrector pili muscles and so is able to demonstrate the characteristic "goose bumps." Goose bumps cease to appear in areas which have received electrology treatment because the arrector pili muscles have been destroyed.

Tertiary hair of the scalp thins with age, or in cases where the patient has excess amounts of the male hormone testosterone. Some experts believe that these people will eventually bald and the tertiary hairs on other areas of the body will become longer, thicker, and more pigmented. This patient will often ask the electrologist to thin or remove the excess hair.

HAIR GROWTH CYCLE

Normal, average growth varies with the type and location of the hair, as well as with the sex of the individual. The hair on the scalp grows at the average rate of ½" (1.25 cm) per month. Hairs around the margin, or hairline, grow very slowly. All hair growth slows with age.

The Life of the Follicle

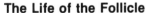

Each follicle produces hair for a varying length of time. The follicle then slows production, and finally goes into a resting state. These cycles are known as **anagen** *(AN ah jen)* **catagen** *(CAHT ah jen)*, and **telogen** *(TEL oh jen)*.

Anagen. The first phase of hair growth is the formation of the hair root. Germinative cells multiply and a column of specialized cells becomes evident. This column will continue to develop into the follicle itself. The papilla develops, followed by the bulb, and hair cell generation begins.

It is at this phase of hair growth that electrology treatments are the most successful. This is because the hair is straight and close to the surface.

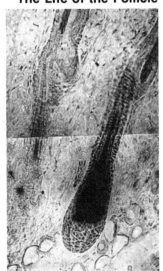

A young follicle just starting to produce a hair. Note bed-hairs of previous cycles which have not been brushed or combed out.

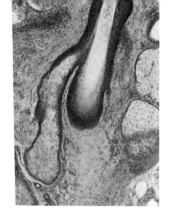

A "bed-hair" is an old follicle. The follicle has shortened past its sebaceous gland.

Catagen. After a period of growth, the catagen phase will begin. The length of time of the growth will depend on many factors such as age, sex, hormone distribution, etc. The papilla first separates from the bulb at the hair root. Nourishment is then decreased, and production of germinal cells slows. The follicle walls begin to shrink, and to dehydrate.

This phase is usually very brief, and sometimes a new hair can be forming while the old hair is still in the follicle. These old hairs are commonly called bed hairs or club hairs. *Waiting to fall out*

Telogen. When the catagen stage is complete, the follicle usually rests until it is stimulated to begin a new cycle. This new phase is the telogen phase. It can be distinguished by the appearance of the bottom of an epilated hair. Often, the club-shaped bulb is attached and can be seen. Additionally, the hair from inside the follicle has a shriveled appearance.

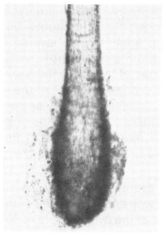

A typical "shed-hair" illustrating club end.

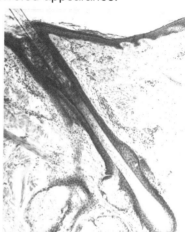

An old hair in a dying follicle.

The success rate of electrology is lowered by those hairs treated in the telogen stage. The hair at this phase is already detached from the papilla, so it will slip very easily from the follicle. The electrologist may think that the hair has been effectively treated, but the lower portion of the follicle will not be destroyed. For this reason, it is best to treat hair in the anagen phase, and impress upon clients the importance of maintaining their appointment schedule.

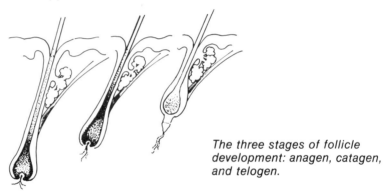

The three stages of follicle development: anagen, catagen, and telogen.

CHARACTERISTICS OF HAIR TEXTURE

The **hand** or feel of the hair is how texture is usually judged. The texture of the hair can also be determined by its appearance, manageability, and the way it reacts to trimming, brushing, combing, etc. The texture is also determined by the mass of the cortex, whether it is fine, medium, or coarse. This must be considered by the electrologist when determining the size of the needle for effective treatment.

Porosity

Porosity *(po ROS i tee)* is the ability of the hair to absorb moisture through the cuticle. Porosity is seldom of concern to the electrologist, unless the hair is so damaged that it breaks during treatment. This would give the false impression of effective treatment, but would result in "regrowth."

Elasticity

Elasticity *(EE las TIS i tee)* is the ability of the hair to stretch and then return to its normal form without breaking. Normal hair is capable of being stretched about one-fifth of its length, and will spring back when released. Elasticity is important to the electrologist only in that it indicates that there is adequate moisture for effective treatment.

Condition

The **condition** of the hair is a complex characteristic that results from many factors. It is of little importance to the electrologist except to note that a sudden appearance of poor condition may be a symptom of a body imbalance. In that instance the electrologist would offer service to the client by advising them to seek medical treatment.

QUESTIONS FOR REVIEW

1. What are the functions of hair?
2. What are the structures related to the hair?
3. Illustrate the structure of an individual hair.
4. What are the three trypes of hair and where are they located?
5. What are the growth cycles of the hair? How are they important?
6. What are the characteristics of the hair?

Chapter 16 Basic Disorders of the Skin

LEARNING OBJECTIVES

Successful mastery of the material in this chapter will be indicated when you can:

1. Define **dermatology.**
2. Describe the skin conditions of erythema and edema.
3. List the principle skin lesions.
4. Define at least 10 common terms applied to disease.
5. Explain what disorders of the sebaceous gland do not prevent electrology treatment.
6. Explain how disorders of the sudoriferous gland affect electrology treatment.
7. Explain how a patient with inflammations is treated.
8. Explain what may cause the appearance of brown spots or freckles during an electrology treatment.
9. Describe correct procedure when a change in a hypertrophy is noted.
10. Name the three types of skin cancer.
11. Describe the post-treatment skin conditions the patient can cause.

INTRODUCTION

Electrologists must learn to recognize skin disorders and deal with them correctly in the office. A patient with inflamed or irritated skin should not be treated, and a patient with an abnormal skin condition may need the permission of a physician before electrology treatments can be given.

It is the electrologist's duty to safeguard the health of the patient by suggesting that the patient see a dermatologist before a skin condition worsens. If a patient refuses to accept the electrologist's advice, it is better to lose the patient than to take the risk of treatment.

In recent years, some dermatologists have added electrologists to their staffs. More often, however, dermatologists refer their hirsute patients to reputable electrologists. It is therefore a good idea to develop a good rapport with local dermatologists and physicians.

DERMATOLOGY DEFINED

The following are terms the electrologist should know:

Dermatology *(dur mah TOL ah jee)* is the study of skin—its nature, structure and functions, diseases and treatment.

A **Dermatologist** *(dur mah TOL ah jist)* is a skin specialist.

Pathology *(pah THOL o jee)* is the study of disease.

Trichology *(tri KOL o jee)* is the study of the hair—its diseases, and care.

Etiology *(ee ti OL oh jee)* is the study of the causes of disease.

Diagnosis *(deye ag NOS sis)* is the recognition of a disease from its symptoms.

Prognosis *(prog NOH sis)* is the foretelling of the probable course of a disease.

In order for the electrologist to recognize skin conditions that may require the attention of a dermatologist, it is important for him or her to understand some of the basic terms and concepts of dermatology. For example, we refer to normal skin as skin clear of all defects. Abnormalities of the skin may include blisters, pimples, eruptions, and rashes.

A **symptom** *(SIMP tom)* is a sign of disease. The symptoms of diseases of the skin are divided into two groups as follows:

1. **Subjective** *(sub JEK tiv)* refers to symptoms that can be felt, such as itching, burning, or pain.
2. **Objective** *(ob JEK tiv)* refers to symptoms that can be seen, such as pimples, pustules, or inflammation.

SKIN CONDITIONS

The epidermis of the skin is composed of living cells, melanin (color pigment), and keratin. The term **keratosis** *(ker ah TOH sis)* refers to a skin condition that results from an excess of keratin. The following are terms that also apply to conditions of the skin:

1. **Hyperkeratosis** *(heye per KER ah TOH sis)* refers to an abnormal increase in the horny layer of the skin. A callus is an example of this condition.
2. **Parakeratosis** *(PAHR ah ker ah TOH sis)* refers to nuclei in the cells of the horny layer of the skin.
3. **Acanthosis** *(ak an THOH sis)* is a condition that is the result of an increased number of prickle cells.
4. **Dyskeratosis** *(DIS ker ah TOH sis)* refers to the imperfect keratinization of individual epidermal cells.
5. **Spongiosis** *(spun jee OH sis)* is a condition that produces a sponge-like appearance of the skin due to an increase of fluid in the cell layers.
6. **Pruritus** *(pruu REYE tis)* is the medical term for a skin inflammation that causes itching.
7. **Erythema** *(er i THEE mah)* is the medical term for redness of the skin.
8. **Edema** *(eh DEE mah)* is the medical term for swelling.
9. **Acute** *(ah CYOOT)* means severe.
10. **Chronic** *(KRON ik)* means long-term or even lifelong.

LESIONS OF THE SKIN

A **lesion** *(LEE zhun)* is a structural change in tissue caused by injury or disease. There are three types of lesions: primary, secondary, and tertiary. The electrologist is concerned with primary and secondary lesions only.

Knowing the principal skin lesions will allow you to distinguish between conditions that affect electrology treatments.

Primary Lesions

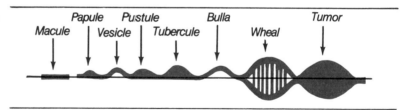

Primary lesions are the first clinically recognizable signs of a skin disease.

1. **Macule** *(MAK yool)*—a small, discolored spot or patch on the surface of the skin, neither raised nor sunken, such as a freckle.
2. **Papule** *(PAP yool)*—a small, elevated pimple in the skin. It contains no fluid, but may develop pus.
3. **Wheal** *(hweel)*—an itchy, swollen lesion that lasts only a few hours. Hives, or the bite of an insect such as a mosquito, are good examples.
4. **Tubercule** *(TOO ber kel)*—a solid lump, larger than a papule. It can project above the surface, lie within, or lie under the skin. It can vary in size from a pea to a walnut.
5. **Tumor** *(TOO mor)*—an external swelling. Tumors can vary in size, shape, and color.
6. **Vesicle** *(VES i kel)*—a blister containing clear fluid. A vesicle can lie within or just beneath the epidermis. The reaction to poison ivy produces small vesicles.
7. **Bulla** *(BUL ah)*—a blister containing watery fluid, similar to a vesicle, but larger.
8. **Pustule** *(PUS chool)*—an elevation of the skin which has an inflamed base and contains pus.

Secondary Lesions

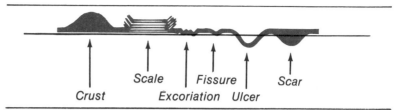

The secondary lesions are those in the skin which develop in the later stages of disease. They are:

1. **Scale** *(skayl)*—an accumulation of epidermal flakes. Scales can be dry or greasy, such as abnormal or excessive dandruff.
2. **Crust** *(krust)*—an accumulation of serum and pus, mixed perhaps with epidermal material. The scab on a sore is an example.

3. **Excoriation** *(ik SKOHR ee ay shun)*—a skin sore or abrasion produced by scratching or scraping. The raw surface due to the loss of the superficial skin after an injury is an example.
4. **Fissure** *(FISH yoor)*—a crack in the skin penetrating into the dermis, as in the case of the chapped hands or lips.
5. **Ulcer** *(UL ser)*—an open lesion on the skin or mucous membrane of the body, accompanied by pus and loss of skin depth.
6. **Scar** *(skahr)*—hardened tissue which forms over injuries that penetrate the dermis.
7. **Stain** *(stayn)*—an abnormal discoloration remaining after the disappearance of moles, freckles or liver spots, sometimes apparent after certain diseases.

DEFINITIONS OF COMMON TERMS APPLIED TO DISEASE

Before describing the disease of the skin so that they may be recognized by the electrologist, it is important to give an understanding of the term **disease.**

Disease *(di ZEEZ)* is any departure from normal health.

Skin disease *(skin di ZEEZ)* is an infection of the skin characterized by an objective lesion (one which can be seen), which may consist of scales, pimples, or pustules.

Acute disease *(ah CYOOT di ZEEZ)* is manifested by symptoms of a more or less violent character and of short duration.

Chronic disease is of long duration, usually mild but recurring.

Infectious disease *(in FEK shus di ZEEZ)* is due to pathogenic germs taken into the body.

Contagious disease *(kahn TAY jus di ZEEZ)* is communicable by contact.

Congenital disease *(cahn JEEN i tahl di ZEEZ)* is present in an infant at birth.

Seasonal disease *(SEE zoh nahl di ZEEZ)* is influenced by the weather, as prickly heat in the summer, and forms of eczema which are more prevalent in cold weather.

Occupational disease, *(ok yoo PAY suh nohl di ZEEZ)* such as dermatitis, is due to certain kinds of employment, and is caused by coming in contact with cosmetics, chemicals, etc.

Parasitic disease *(par ah SIT ik di ZEEZ)* is caused by vegetable or animal parasites, such as pediculosis or ringworm.

Pathogenic disease *(path o JEN ik di ZEEZ)* is produced by disease-producing bacteria such as staphylococus and streptococcus, which are pus-forming bacteria.

Systemic disease *(si STEM ik di ZEEZ)* is due to under or overfunctioning of the internal glands. It may be caused by diet.

Venereal disease *(ve NEER ee al di ZEEZ)* is a contagious disease which is contracted during sexual intercourse with an infected person.

Epidemic *(ep i DEM ik)* is the manifestation of a disease that attacks a large number of people, within one locality, simultaneously. Infantile paralysis, influenza, virus, or smallpox are examples of epidemic-causing diseases.

Allergy *(AL er jee)* is a sensitivity which certain people develop to normally harmless substances. Skin allergies are quite common. Contact with certain types of cosmetics, medicines, tints, or eating certain foods all may bring out an itching eruption, accompanied by redness, swelling, blisters, oozing and scaling.

Inflammation *(in fla MAY shun)* is a sign of skin disorder characterized by redness, pain, swelling and heat.

NOTE: *The terms **infectious disease, communicable disease,** and **contagious disease** are often used interchangeably.*

CAUTION: *Do not perform an electrology treatment on any skin disorder that has symptoms of inflammation, edema, or open lesions.*

DISORDERS OF THE SEBACEOUS GLANDS

There are several common disorders of the sebaceous (oil) glands which the electrologist should be able to identify. Patients with the following disorders may safely receive electrology treatments as long as the particular disorder is not severe.

Pimples

Pimples *(PIMP pels)* occur when the follicle becomes filled with oil, dead cells and bacteria. It often swells and ruptures, causing the debris to escape into the dermis, resulting in irritation and inflammation. White blood cells rush in to fight the bacteria and create a material called **pus,** a sticky, yellowish secretation. In the beginning, a pimple appears as an inflamed, red or blue-red lump.

When the overtaxed follicle ruptures near the surface of the skin it is not serious, and will usually heal rapidly, leaving no permanent mark. If the follicle breaks deep underneath the skin, however, the pimple will be more severe, take longer to heal, and may leave permanent scars.

Comedones

Comedones *(kom eh DON neez),* or blackheads, are wormlike masses of keratinized cells and hardened sebum appearing most frequently on the face, chest, shoulders, and back.

When the hair follicle is filled with an excess of oil from the sebaceous glands and an accumulation of dead cells, a blackhead forms, creating a blockage at the mouth of the hair follicle. If this condition becomes severe, the patient should seek medical attention.

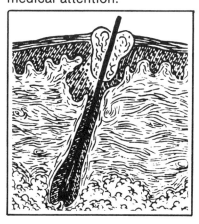

Blackhead (plug of sebaceous matter and dead cells) forming around the mouth of hair follicle.

Milia   Milia *(MIL ee ah),* or whiteheads, are a disorder of the sebaceous (oil) glands caused by the accumulation of dead cells and sebum trapped beneath the skin. This may occur on any part of the face, and occasionally on the chest, shoulders and back. Whiteheads look like small grains of sand under the skin.

Acne   Acne *(AK nee)* is a chronic inflammatory disorder of the skin, usually related to hormonal changes and overactive sebaceous glands during adolescence. Common acne is also known as acne simplex or acne vulgaris.

Acne types range from noncontagious pimples to deep-seated skin conditions. Though acne generally starts at the onset of puberty, it can also afflict adults.

Modern studies show that acne is often due to heredity, but that the condition can be aggravated by emotional stress and environmental factors. Acne is not caused by any particular food, drink, or personal habit.

Acne is accompanied by blackheads, pustules, and pimples that are red, swollen, and contain pus. The pus is seen as a yellowish or white-tinged center in some blemishes. In more advanced cases of acne, cysts appear. Cysts are red swollen bumps beneath the skin.

Seborrhea   Seborrhea *(seb o REE ah)* is a skin condition caused by overactivity of the sebaceous glands. An oily or shiny condition of the nose, forehead or scalp indicates the presence of seborrhea. It is detected on the scalp by unusual amounts of oil on the hair. Seborrhea is often the basis of an acne condition.

Rosacea   Rosacea *(roh ZAY shee ah)* is associated with excessive oiliness of the skin, chronic redness, dilation of the blood vessels, and the formation of papules and pustules. The skin becomes coarse and the pores enlarged.

Steatoma   Steatoma *(stee ah TOH mah)* or wen is a subcutaneous tumor of the sebaceous glands. It ranges in size from a pea to an orange and consists of sebum. It usually occurs on the scalp, neck or back.

Asteatosis   Asteatosis *(As tee ah TOH sis)* is a condition of dry, scaly skin, characterized by deficiency of sebum. Asteatosis is usually due to aging or bodily disorders. In local conditions, it may be caused by alkalies, such as those found in soap.

Furuncle   Furuncle *(FU rung kel),* also called a boil, is caused by bacteria that enter the skin through the hair follicles. It is a subcutaneous abscess that fills with pus. A boil can be painful and should be treated by a physician.

THE SEBACEOUS GLAND

SEBACEOUS GLAND FUNCTIONING IN A NORMAL MANNER

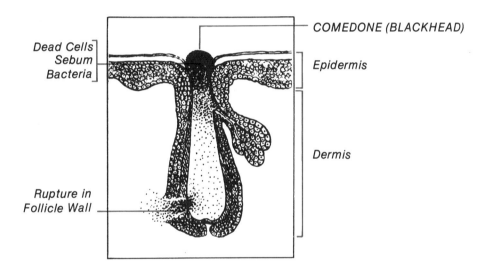

Epidermis

Discharged Sebum

Sebaceous Duct

Sebaceous Gland

Follicle

COMEDONE (BLACKHEAD)

Dead Cells
Sebum
Bacteria

Epidermis

Dermis

Rupture in
Follicle Wall

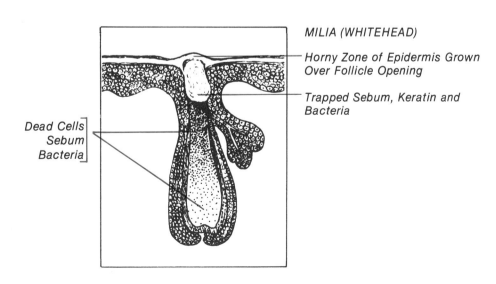

MILIA (WHITEHEAD)

Horny Zone of Epidermis Grown Over Follicle Opening

Trapped Sebum, Keratin and Bacteria

Dead Cells
Sebum
Bacteria

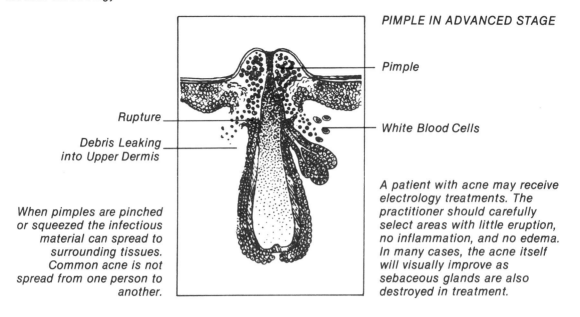

PIMPLE IN ADVANCED STAGE

Pimple

Rupture

White Blood Cells

Debris Leaking
into Upper Dermis

When pimples are pinched or squeezed the infectious material can spread to surrounding tissues. Common acne is not spread from one person to another.

A patient with acne may receive electrology treatments. The practitioner should carefully select areas with little eruption, no inflammation, and no edema. In many cases, the acne itself will visually improve as sebaceous glands are also destroyed in treatment.

DISORDERS OF THE SUDORIFEROUS GLANDS

Patients with disorders of the sudoriferous glands may safely receive electrology treatments. Disorders of this type pose no threat to the health of the electrologist working on the afflicted patient.

Bromidrosis *(BROH mi DROH sis)* or **Osmidrosis** *(oz mi DROH sis)* refers to foul-smelling perspiration, usually noticeable in the armpits or on the feet.

Anidrosis *(an i DROH sis)* or lack of perspiration, is often a result of fever or certain skin diseases. Anidrosis requires medical treatment.

Hyperidrosis *(HEYE per i DROH sis)* or excessive perspiration, is caused by intense heat or general body weakness. The most commonly affected parts are the armpits, joints and feet. Hyperidrosis also requires medical attention.

Miliaria rubra *(mil ee AIR ee uh ROOHB rah)* or prickly heat, is an acute inflammation of the sweat glands characterized by small, red vesicles and accompanied by burning and itching of the skin. It is caused by exposure to excessive heat and obesity.

INFLAMMATIONS

Dermatitis *(dur mah TEYE tis)* is a term used to denote an inflammatory condition of the skin, caused by allergy. The lesions come in various forms, such as vesicles and papules. Electrologists may give treatment around, but not directly on, these lesions. If possible, avoid the use of any aftertreatment product that may further irritate the area.

Eczema *(EK ze mah)* is an inflammatory condition of the skin, either acute or chronic in nature, presenting many forms of dry or moist lesions. It is frequently accompanied by itching, burning and various other unpleasant sensations. All cases of eczema should be referred to a physician for treatment. Eczema may be the result of some type of allergy or internal disorder.

The term **eczema** is applied to any number of surface lesions of the skin. It is usually a red, blistered, oozing area that itches painfully. Because of the painful nature of this inflammation, patients will probably not request electrology treatments until the disorder clears or lessens.

Psoriasis *(so REYE ah sis)* is a common, chronic, inflammatory skin disease whose cause is unknown. It is usually found on the scalp, elbows, knees, chest and lower back, rarely on the face. The lesions are round, dry patches covered with coarse, silvery scales. If irritated, bleeding points occur. While not contagious, this disorder can spread by irritating it. Patients with psoriasis may receive electrology treatments as long as the lesions are not directly touched.

Herpes simplex *(HUR peez SIM pleks)* is a viral infection of unknown origin. It is characterized by the eruption of a single group of vesicles on a red, swollen base. The blisters may appear on the face or genital area. Electrology treatment should be restricted to those areas of the body not affected by the disease in order to avoid spreading the disease.

CAUTION: *Herpes is extremely contagious and some authorities feel that as long as any blisters appear on the body, all treatment should be avoided.*

Impetigo *(im pe TEE goh)* is a highly contagious skin disease which chiefly affects children. During the active stage of the disease, oozing lesions appear daily and spread. Lesions appear on the hands, face and legs, characterized by a light brown crust. It is not advisable to work on patients with impetigo as the disease may be transferred to other parts of the patient's body or even to the electrologist.

PIGMENTATIONS OF THE SKIN

In abnormal circumstances, pigment may come from inside or outside the body. Abnormal colors are seen in every skin disorder and many systemic disorders. Changes in pigmentation are observed when certain drugs are being taken internally. Abnormal pigmentation will not interfere greatly with electrology treatment. You should be aware that the appearance of brown spots and freckles during the electrology treatment may be a sign of overtreatment of an area. Some patients hyperpigmentate easily, especially those with dark or black skin. It may take from several months to two years for hyperpigmentation to disappear.

Lentigines *(len TIJ i neez)* (singular, Lentigo), or freckles, are small yellowish to brownish colored spots on parts of the body exposed to sunlight and air.

Stains *(staynz)* are abnormal brown skin patches, having an irregular circular shape. Their permanent color is due to the presence of blood pigment. They occur during aging, after certain diseases, and after the appearance of moles, freckles and liver spots. The cause of stains is unknown.

Chloasma *(kloh AZ mah)* is characterized by increased deposits of pigment in the skin. It is found mainly on the forehead, nose and cheeks. Chloasma is also called *moth patches* or *liver spots.*

Naevus *(NEE vuhs),* or birthmarks, are malformations of the skin due to pigmentation or dilated capillaries. Many times a naevus will be very hairy. Birthmarks are present on the skin at birth. Some birthmarks are known to regress or disappear with time. In some cases, a physician may advise plastic surgery or a tattoo method to conceal the birthmark.

Leucoderma *(LOO koh DER mah)* refers to abnormal light patches of skin due to congenital pigmentation. Leucoderma may be classified in the following ways:

1. Vitiligo *(vit i LEE goh)*—an acquired condition of leucoderma affecting the skin or the hair in patches.
2. Albinism *(AL bi niz em)*—a congenital absence of melanin pigment in the body, including the skin, hair and eyes. The hair is silky and white. The skin is pinkish white and will not tan.

CAUTION: *Color changes, a crack on the skin, thickening or discoloration ranging from shades of red to brown and purple to almost black, may be danger signals and should be examined by a dermatologist.*

HYPERTROPHIES (NEW GROWTHS)

A **hypertrophy** *(heye PUR trah fee)* is an excessive growth.

Keratoma *(ker ah TOH mah)*, or callus, is a thickened patch of epidermis, caused by friction, usually on the hands and feet. Hair does not usually grow in areas affected by keratoma so the electrologist will probably not have to work on those areas.

A **mole** *(mohl)* is a small, brown spot on the skin. Moles are believed to be inherited. They range in color from pale tan to brown or bluish black. Some moles are small and flat, resembling freckles. Others are more deeply seated and darker in color. Large, dark terminal hairs often occur in moles.

CAUTION: *Any change in a mole requires medical attention as it may be a sign of malignancy. If a patient requests electrology treatment of a hairy mole, have them obtain formal permission from a physician. This will protect you legally from any law suits that may arise from the treatment of the mole. Although there are no recorded problems with moles stemming from electrology treatment, this is still a controversial area. Do not pluck hair from moles.*

Verruca *(ve ROO kah)* is the technical term for wart. It is a viral infection of the epidermis. Warts can spread from one location to another, particularly along a scratch in the skin. They may be found on various parts of the body, but appear most often on the hands and fingers. Warts are contagious and should not be treated by the electrologist.

Keloids *(KEE loids)* are raised masses of fibrous scar tissue. They are an abnormal reaction to injury of the skin. Certain races are prone to keloids; they appear frequently on black skin. Electrologists should note when patients have existing keloids in order to avoid overtreating the hair follicles and causing more keloids.

NOTE: *It would be wise to have a keloidal patient sign a release before electrology treatment is begun. Patients with keloids should always be given a treatment test to assess the skin's reaction to electrology before regular treatments are given.*

OTHER SERIOUS DISORDERS OF THE SKIN

Skin Cancer

Other serious skin disorders the electrologist should be familiar with are skin cancer, tumors, and veneral disease.

There are three kinds of skin cancer. The least malignant and most common is **Basal cell carcinoma.** This type of cancer is characterized by light or pearly nodules and visible blood vessels.

Squamous cell carcinoma is different in appearance from the basal, or basic, type. It consists of scaly, red papules. Blood vessels are not visible. This cancer is more serious than the Basal cell carcinoma.

The most serious skin cancer is the **Malignant melanoma.** This cancer is characterized by dark (brown, black, or discolored) patches on the skin. Unlike moles, these patches are usually hairless and irregular in shape.

The electrologist should not attempt to diagnose lumps, lesions, ulcerations, or discoloration as skin cancer, but should be able to recognize serious skin disorders and suggest that the client seek medical attention without delay.

Tumors

Tumors *(TOO mors)* are abnormal growths of swollen tissue that can be located on any part of the body. Some tumors are benign (mild in character and not likely to recur after removal) which means they are not harmful. Some tumors are malignant and are more serious as they can recur after removal.

Venereal Diseases

Venereal *(ve NEER ee al)* diseases are those associated with the sexual organs and are characterized by **chancre** *(SHANG ker)* sores and rashes on the skin. **Syphilis** *(SIF i lis)* is a serious disease transmitted through sexual contact with an infected person. When any sore, especially a sore that is hard and lacerated (with a hole in the center) first appears, a physician should be consulted. Without treatment the sore may go away only to appear later in the form of a rash. This is secondary syphilis. The condition may then become latent (present but not visible). Secondary syphilis can cause degeneration of various body parts, and ultimately causes death. Gonorrhea is a more common disease than syphilis, characterized by a discharge and burning sensation when urinating. If left untreated, harmful bacteria can enter the bloodstream.

Electrologists should treat patients with venereal disease only after they have signed a release. Treatment should then only be given to those areas not affected by the sores, lacerations or rashes induced by the disorder. Some authorities feel that patients with visible herpes simplex sores should not be treated until the sores have disappeared.

POST-TREATMENT SKIN DISORDERS

There are several types of skin disorders that may occur after a patient receives an electrology treatment. These may be directly related to the treatments themselves or may be a result or poor aftertreatment care by the patient at home.

Overtreatment

Overtreatment of an area can produce keloids (as discussed earlier), scaly skin, pitting, scarring, or ruptured capillaries. For a full discussion on the effects of maltreatment, see Chapter 6.

Other Sources

Patients can cause infection in treated areas by scratching, picking at scabs, or applying cosmetics to healing follicles. They can also transfer infection by touching an infected part of the body and then touching the treatment area.

Demographia *(dem oh GRAF ee ah)*. This is a temporary condition in which the patient experiences swelling due to scratching or friction on the skin. The electrology patient will have to decide whether they wish to endure the temporary swelling that will occur after every electrology treatment.

Folliculitis. *(foh lik yoo LEYE tis)*. Occasionally, treated hair follicles will become slightly infected and pustules will appear. These pustules will develop scabs which drop off in a few days time. If the skin is not cared for properly at this point the infection will go deeper, becoming a condition called folliculitis. Severe folliculitis can cause pitting. Folliculitis may also be caused by ingrown hairs or by the application of cosmetics directly upon the areas which have just received electrology treatments.

Some patients may be allergic to electrology treatments. This occurs when the patient develops an allergy to galvanic lye. The electrologist can often remedy this situation by switching from the galvanic method to the shortwave method of electrology.

QUESTIONS FOR REVIEW

1. What is dermatology?
2. What is erythema? Edema?
3. What are the principle skin lesions?
4. What are 10 common terms applied to disease?
5. What disorders of the sebaceous gland do not prevent electrology treatment?
6. How do disorders of the sudoriferous gland affect electrology treatment?
7. How is a patient with inflammations treated?
8. What may cause the appearance of brown spots or freckles during an electrology treatment?
9. What is the correct procedure when a change in a hypertrophy is noted?
10. What are the three types of skin cancer?
11. What post-treatment skin conditions can the patient cause?

Chapter 17 The Skin—Nutrition, Aging and Surgery

LEARNING OBJECTIVES

Successful mastery of the material in this chapter will be indicated when you can:

1. List the three basic food elements and explain why they are important to overall health.
2. List the four basic food groups.
3. Describe two ways in which aging skin makes electrology treatment more difficult.
4. Explain how air pollution harms skin.
5. Explain how scar tissue can affect electrology treatment.

INTRODUCTION

Skin is affected by nutrition, aging and cosmetic surgery. When any of these factors affect your patient's skin, they will influence the electrology treatment you give. Nutrition also affects hair growth, especially on anorexic or obese patients (see Chapter 13 for a detailed discussion on the causes of excess hair growth).

NUTRITION

The skin is nourished by the blood and lymphatic systems of the body. A major part of the circulatory system is devoted to the nourishment of the skin. Essential nutrients for growth, maintenance, and repair are circulated through the skin by blood and lymph. Numerous networks of arteries, capillaries, and lymphatics beneath the skin supply nutrients to the glands and tissues. Good nutrition helps the skin to function normally. Allergies, rashes, and other disorders of the skin are often the result of poor nutrition.

Food Elements

When your patient's skin is in poor condition and you suspect inadequate nutrition, you may help your client by discussing the benefits of a well-balanced diet and the three basic food elements. They are fats, carbohydrates, and proteins.

Fats are important to the body because they enable the sebaceous glands to produce certain materials which help to lubricate the skin.

Carbohydrates include all the various types of sugars, starches, gums, pectins, and cellulose. The most important carbohydrate is glucose. It provides most of the body's energy.

Proteins are essential to life. All living things are composed of proteins. Protein is composed of amino acids, some of which the body can produce and others of which must be obtained from food. Those obtained from food are called *essential amino acids.* When an essential amino acid is missing from the diet, specific deficiency symptoms such as weight loss, anemia, and lowered resistance to infection and injury to organs begin to develop.

Dieting

When we cut our food intake for the purpose of losing weight, we also cut down on the intake of minerals and vitamins which help to keep the entire body healthy. When weight is reduced too fast, the skin will sag and wrinkle rather than gradually return to its former condition. Crash diets should not be undertaken without the supervision of a physician as the entire body, especially the skin, will suffer.

Nutrition Essentials for Skin Health

An individual's nutritional needs depend on such factors as age, physical build, and amount of activity. Your patient may benefit from a knowledge of the four basic food groups. These groups should be selected from to promote a balanced diet. The four groups are: dairy, meat and protein, vegetable-fruit, and bread-cereal.

Dairy Group

Milk is good for growth and for strong bones. It should be included in the daily diet unless a physician recommends otherwise to, for example, people who need to control their intake of cholesterol. Other dairy products include yogurt, cheese and butter.

Children—2 to 3 cups
Teenagers—4 or more cups
Adults—2 or more cups

Meat and Protein Alternatives Group

Good sources of protein are beef, veal, pork, lamb, organ meats, fish, poultry, and alternatives such as nuts, peas, beans and eggs.

Two or more servings daily.

Vegetable-Fruit Group

Fruits and vegetables are important sources of vitamins C and A. Fruits and vegetables, raw or cooked, should be eaten every day.

Four more servings daily.

Bread-Cereal Group

Whole grain cereal is best. Serving size may very with the individual's age, activity, and body build. The main consideration is to provide the body with a well-balanced diet for maximum nutrition and health maintenance.

Four or more servings daily.

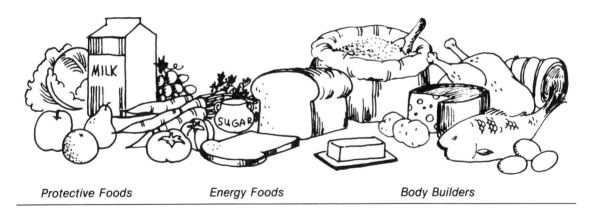

Protective Foods	Energy Foods	Body Builders

When studying nutrition, it is important to remember that water is essential to life. Water makes up one-half to two-thirds of the human body. It aids digestion, carries waste materials from the body, helps to form body fluids, sustains the health of all cells, helps regulate the temperature of the body, and much more. It is easy to see that drinking enough water will help keep the skin healthy and attractive.

Skin as an Indicator of Health

We know that skin derives its nourishment from the bloodstream, and that a well-balanced diet provides the nutrients essential to keeping the skin healthy and attractive. The skin reveals much about the body, and essential nutrients it may lack. For example, a lack of vitamin C over a period of time can cause **scurvy** *(SKUR vee)*, a disease that produces skin lesions. **Pellagra** *(peh LAHG rah)*, a result of a severe vitamin B deficiency which shows a characteristic skin rash that can cause scarring. Other deficiencies that can have a nutritional origin are such skin disorders as acne, eczema, psoriasis, and dermatitis (for a complete discussion on skin disorders, see Chapter 15).

Changes in the color of the skin can also be an indication of the body's nutritional state. This is due to changes in the color of the blood beneath the surface of the skin. A pale, dry skin may indicate anemia. Severe protein and calorie deficiency in children causes characteristic changes in skin and hair color. Jaundice is characterized by a yellowish cast to the skin.

The skin is an indicator of any number of minor or serious internal problems. Liver disease will cause a yellowish cast in the skin and redness of the palms of the hands. Yellow or white fatty papules around the eyes may indicate an elevated cholesterol level, which can cause heart problems. Any chronic itching, sudden change in skin color or growth that appears should be checked by a dermatologist.

Tobacco, alcohol, and drugs can contribute to the premature aging of skin.

AGING   Usually around the ages of 40 or 50, men and women find that fine lines and wrinkles on the face and neck become more prominent. Loss of the skin's elasticity and the onset of biological changes at midlife contribute to this process. Aging skin can make electrology treatments more difficult. Skin which is soft and saggy, for example, will make proper insertion of the electrology needle more difficult than firm skin would. Dryness, a characteristic of aging skin, is a deterrent in proper electrology treatment. This is because moisture (from water as opposed to oils) is needed for electric current to destroy tissue. These patients generally feel treatment less and are able to withstand higher intensities, due to the decrease in moisture content of the skin.

Effects of Excessive Sunlight   Overexposure to the sun is harmful to the skin. People whose skins have been overexposed during their younger years generally start to show signs of age between the ages of 38 and 45. This is partially due to structural damage that affects the skin's elasticity. Once the skin has lost its elasticity, it cannot be restored. People who sunbathe should always apply a screening oil or lotion before exposure. Patients with severe sunburn should be referred to a physician.

Air Pollution   The chemical reactions of pollutants can be devastating to the skin. Sulphur-containing compounds are among the most common pollutants in the air. When polluted air contacts the skin, it partially converts to sulfuric acid. The dehydration that results is harmful to the skin. Areas of the body that are protected by clothing remain looking younger longer, but the face, hands, and other areas constantly exposed age more rapidly.

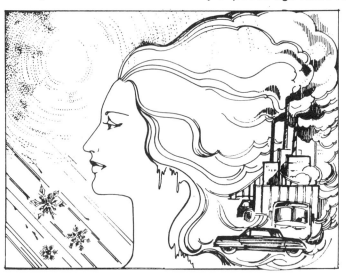

The face in direct contact with environmental enemies of the skin. These enemies include overexposure to the sun, harsh weather conditions, pollution in the air. Emollients, creams or lotions can help protect the skin from these environmental enemies.

Excessive Massage   Massage is good for the skin if done properly and professionally. However, constant rubbing, pulling, or incorrect massage can weaken collagen fibers, resulting in wrinkles. Advise the patient to use gentle, upward movements when cleansing the skin. Tugging, pulling on, or pushing the facial muscles should be avoided. Facial exercises that include exaggerated facial expressions may contribute to premature wrinkling and lining of the skin. Biting the inside of the cheeks, and pursing or biting the lips, should also be avoided.

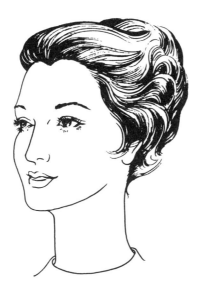

People who guard their health and give the skin daily care will retain a youthful appearance longer. It is usually around the age of 35 that fine expression lines begin to appear around the eyes, the mouth and on the forehead. Women can use subtle makeup to conceal the signs of aging, but too much makeup will only call attention to lines in the face.

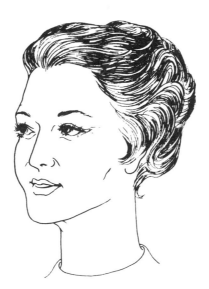

By 45 years of age the expression patterns on most faces begin to deepen around the mouth, the eyes and on the forehead. The skin shows loss of elasticity, especially around the eyes. A double chin may start to show and the neck may begin to appear crepy in texture.

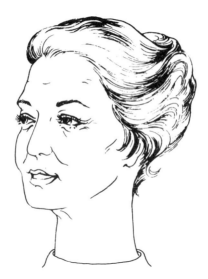

By the age of 55 the skin becomes looser and the folds and sagging tissue around the eyes will be more pronounced. The cheek bones appear to be more prominent and the naso-labial (nose to mouth) folds will be more distinct. An overweight person will likely notice the formation of a double chin.

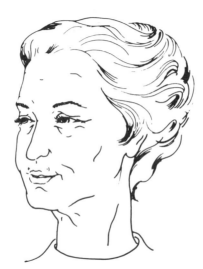

As we age, the skull may remain the same or start to shrink while the skin continues to grow. This causes the skin to sag. By age 65 to 70, the contour of the face changes and there are deeper folds and lines due to loss of muscle tone. The cheeks and jaws become flabby and the nose and chin usually appear to be more prominent. Drooping tissue around the eyes cause them to appear smaller. Lines on the neck deepen and skin becomes loose and crepy.

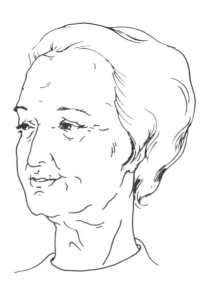

By age 75 and into advanced age, all expression lines and folds in the face deepen. The head shrinks, causing increased sagging of skin and underlying muscles. The small lines that have been forming on the face become more prominent. During advanced age, the aging process continues so that each year the face gradually becomes older looking. Some people become more attractive as they mature as the signs of aging add character and expression to the face. Many popular motion picture, stage and television actors and actresses reach the peak of their careers after they have attained their mature years.

PLASTIC SURGERY Patients who have plastic surgery will have scars. If the incisions are not yet completely healed or appear red or swollen, electrology treatments should of course be avoided in those areas. If the incisions are healed and scar tissue remains, electrology treatment can safely be given on or near the area. Scar tissue will produce distorted hair follicles, however, so proper needle insertion will be made more difficult than usual. If you must work directly on scar tissue, remember to space your insertions a good distance from one another as scar tissue does not heal as easily as normal skin.

Types of Plastic Surgery There are many different types of plastic surgery possibly undergone by the electrology patient which have left scar tissue on the areas you are to treat.

Rhytidectomy *(rit i DEK toh mee)* is the clinical name for a face-lift. Incisions for this procedure are made on the scalp, in front of the ear, around the earlobe and back into the neck hairline.

Blepharolplasty *(BLEF ah roh plas tee)* is the clinical name for eyelid correction. Incisions from this procedure will be found above, below, and at the outside of the eye.

Rhinoplasty *(REYE noh plas tee)* is commonly known as a nose-job. Most of the surgery for this procedure is done inside the nose so the only visible incisions would be at the base of either nostril.

QUESTIONS FOR REVIEW
1. What are the three basic food elements and how are they important to health?
2. What are the four basic food groups?
3. In what two ways does aging skin make electrology treatment more difficult.
4. How does air pollution harm the skin?
5. How can scar tissue affect electrology treatment?

Chapter 18 Image Projection for the Professional Electrologist

LEARNING OBJECTIVES

Successful mastery of the material in this chapter will be indicated when you can:

1. List the areas of healthful living related to personal and public hygiene.
2. Give the benefits of regular exercise.
3. Explain why a healthy attitude is important.
4. List the rules to follow for personal cleanliness and good health.
5. Explain why good posture is important.
6. List the rules for good posture.
7. Describe the proper ways to care for hands and feet.

INTRODUCTION

Good health, personal hygiene, and grooming are requirements for the successful practice of electrology. Without these basic assets, you cannot work efficiently, nor can you enjoy your full potential.

Visual impressions are also important. As a professional electrologist you must always create a good first impression when meeting a patient, and that good first impression should be a lasting one. You cannot create a good visual impression if you have neglected your posture and your physical appearance. It is important to learn to stand, sit, and walk with good posture in order to prevent fatigue, backache, and other discomforts.

HYGIENE

Hygiene deals with healthful living. It includes both personal and public hygiene.

Personal Hygiene

Personal hygiene concerns the intelligent care taken by the individual to preserve health by following the rules of healthful living, especially as they relate to:

1. Cleanliness
2. Oral hygiene
3. Posture
4. Exercise
5. Relaxation
6. Adequate sleep
7. Balanced diet
8. Healthy attitude

Public Hygiene

Public hygiene or **sanitation** refers to the steps which should be taken by the government to promote public health. In order for the government to carry out its responsibilities to protect the health, safety, and welfare of its citizens, steps should be taken to assure:

1. Pure air
2. Pure food
3. Pure water
4. Adequate sewage
5. Control of disease
6. Adequate medical facilities

Hygienic Rules of Living and Good Grooming

Appearance—Keep your appearance at its best giving daily attention to all the important details that help you to present a clean, neat, and attractive appearance.

Daily bath or shower and deodorant—Keep yourself pleasant to be near by taking a daily bath or shower, and using an effective deodorant or antiperspirant when needed. Use cologne and other fragrances sparingly.

Oral hygiene (teeth and breath)—Brush your teeth regularly, especially after meals and at bedtime. Use mouthwash to help eliminate bad breath. Have regular dental and physical checkups.

Hair and makeup (female)—Keep your hair clean and lustrous. Wear an attractive, modern hairstyle that flatters your face and features. Keep your eyebrows well groomed. Never wear makeup that is showy or poorly applied.

Hair, beard and/or mustache—Keep your hair clean and lustrous. Wear an attractive, modern hairstyle. Trim excess hair from nostrils if necessary. If you choose to wear a beard or mustache, keep it styled and trimmed.

Clothing and shoes—Uniforms should be neat, clean, and properly fitted. Select clothes that make the most of your individual body build. Wear fresh undergarments every day. Men should wear clean socks, and women should wear clean pantyhose that are free from runs and wrinkles. Shoes should be kept clean and in perfect condition. They should be comfortable, well fitted, and sensibly styled.

Hands and nails—Hands should be clean at all times and nails well cared for. A woman who prefers colored polish should be sure that it is never smeared or chipped.

MAINTAINING HEALTH AND ATTRACTIVENESS

A poor appearance is often a sign of health problems. Good health is reflected in the skin, eyes, hair, and in the general body functions. The skin is usually the first part of the body to show the effects of neglected health. A healthy person will usually have a clear complexion, luxuriant hair, and bright, clear eyes. Hair and eyes that lack luster and a complexion that is dull are indicative of:

1. Sluggish circulation of the blood due to lack of proper exercise and recreation.
2. Lack of fresh air.

3. Poor eating habits, lack of proper nutrition, and irregular elimination of body wastes.
4. Lack of rest and relaxation, and poor sleeping habits.

Exercise and Recreation Exercise and recreation keep the muscles firm and strong and the entire body in good physical shape. The following are a few of the benefits that result from regular exercise:

1. Exercise helps to circulate blood so that nutrients in food are properly utilized by the body. The blood carries essential nutrients to all parts of the body.
2. A larger supply of oxygen enters the body due to the increased action of the lungs.
3. Recreation and exercise done in the fresh air and sunshine help to supply the body with essential vitamin D. Overexposure to sun should be avoided, however.

Well Balanced Meals Eating well-balanced meals at regular intervals and drinking sufficient amounts of water will keep the digestive system functioning properly. One of the basic causes of poor health is poor diet. It is important to avoid poor eating habits such as:

1. Not eating enough of the right kinds of food. This may lead to weight loss, lowered resistance, or disease. An underweight person who has no appetite and eats too little is not getting proper nutrition.

2. Overeating is hard on the digestive system and on organs of elimination. Eating too many rich and high calorie foods will often lead to excessive weight gain. A person who is very overweight should make every effort to get rid of excess poundage. Such a person should see a physician before starting a diet.

Fatigue Fatigue resulting from work, exercise, mental effort, or the strain caused by hurry and worry, should always be relieved by a period of rest and relaxation. Overextension and lack of rest tend to drain the body of its vitality. Therefore, an adequate amount of sleep, not less than seven hours, is necessary. This allows the body to recover from the fatigue of the day's activities and to reenergize itself. A rested body and mind help to create a sense of well-being.

HEALTHY ATTITUDE The mind and body operate as a unit. A well-balanced condition of body and mind results in good health, which leads to normal functioning. One can develop a healthy attitude through self-control. Worry and fear should be replaced with the health-giving qualities of cheerfulness, courage, and hope. Outside interests and recreation can relieve the strain and monotony of hard work.

Thoughts and Emotions   Thoughts and emotions influence body activities. For example, an angry thought may cause the face to turn red and increase the heart action. A thought may either stimulate or depress the functions of the body. Strong emotions such as worry, anger, and fear, have harmful effects on the heart, arteries, and glands. Mental depression weakens the functions of the organs, thereby lowering the resistance of the body to disease.

REMINDER   *Good grooming adds to self-esteem. Following the rules of hygienic living, cultivating positive attitudes, and keeping the emotions under control will help you to project yourself as a successful electrologist.*

CHECKLIST FOR PERSONAL CLEANLINESS AND GOOD HEALTH

1. Keep the body clean by taking a daily bath or shower.
2. Prevent body odor by using a deodorant, cologne or after shave.
3. Keep teeth and gums in good condition. Brush teeth at least twice daily with a good toothpaste.
4. Have a dental examination every six months.
5. Avoid bad breath by rinsing mouth with good antiseptic.
6. Have tissues handy in case you cough or sneeze.
7. Keep shoes clean and wear clean hose.
8. Wear clean underwear and a clean uniform each day.
9. Keep hair well groomed.
10. Keep hands and nails in good condition.

11. Wash hands before and after treating each patient and after visiting the rest room.
12. Avoid the common use of towels, drinking cups, hairbrushes, and combs.
13. Breathe fresh air. Keep your home and office well ventilated.
14. Drink eight glasses of water each day.
15. Follow a balanced diet.
16. Stand, sit, and walk with good posture.
17. Get enough sleep and relaxation.
18. Participate in recreation and outdoor exercise.
19. Have regular physical examinations.

POSTURE AND A POISED APPEARANCE   Correct posture is vitally important to your body because it helps to prevent fatigue, improves your personal appearance, and permits you to move gracefully in your everyday work as an electrologist.

Good posture is an important part of personal care. Its continued practice assists in the prevention of many physical problems. In addition, it is a self-discipline that contributes to the development of other good habits. These are the determining elements of a gracious and pleasing personality. When present, they indicate a poised and orderly personality.

The electrologist should consider appearance, poise, and personality to be almost as important as technical knowledge and manual skills.

Standing   Regular exercise keeps the muscles of the body in good condition and assists in forming the habit of good posture. Practice trains muscles to hold the body correctly. Good posture is a matter of habit. Avoid slouching, humped shoulders, and spinal curvature while working.

To walk and stand correctly and achieve good body balance, distribute your body weight properly.

People who are on their feet for long hours should stand with their feet close enough together so that the body weight is distributed onto the balls of the feet rather than onto the heels. Standing with the feet side by side tends to throw the body out of alignment, causing fatigue. When one foot is placed slightly in front of the other, the body weight is easier to balance. Good balance, muscle control, and coordination of the hands and feet help to prevent fatigue.

The basic at ease stance for men and women is described as follows. To practice the basic standing position:

1. Turn the left foot out at a 45^0 angle.
2. Point the right foot straight forward, with the heel even with the instep of the left foot. The right foot may also be placed several inches in front of the left. This is usually more comfortable.
3. Keep both knees slightly flexed (flexed knees act as shock absorbers when walking or standing), with the right knee bent inward.

The basic stance enables you to shift your weight from one foot to another easily. Place the left foot forward with the right foot angled when it is more practical to do so.

The basic stance is helpful when you are standing in one position for any length of time because it helps to prevent fatigue. This is especially true when you are talking with people, working at a table filing reports, or performing services. If you make the basic stance an everyday habit, you will keep your entire body in alignment, thus preventing the fatigue, headaches, and backaches that are generally the result of poor posture.

Points for Avoiding   Poor posture—Don't place the feet side by side when it is
Back Strain   necessary to bend over.

Correct posture—Keep the knees flexed when standing.

Comfort for the patient and the electrologist—The electrologist's chair should be adjusted to a height that is comfortable.

POSTURE
IMPROVEMENT
Body Posture

1. Stiff, rigid poor posture
2. Slumped, humped poor posture
3. Swayback or lordosis *(lor DOH sis)*
4. Drooped shoulders or kyphosis *(keye FOH sis)*
5. Swayback and drooped shoulders or scoliosis *(SKOH lee OH sis)*

Correct body posture   *Defective body posture*

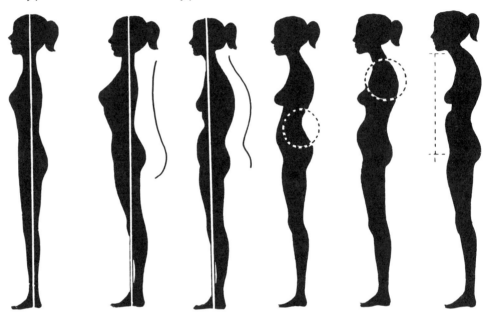

Normal   *1. Stiff*   *2. Slumped*   *3. Lordosis*   *4. Kyphosis*   *5. Scoliosis*

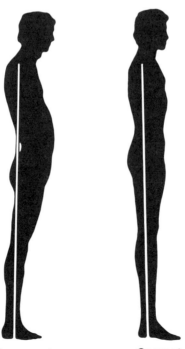

Incorrect   *Correct*

Posture Correction

Use a mirror to note the defects in your posture that need to be corrected. Then observe the following good posture rules:

1. Carry weight on the balls of your feet, not on the heels. Imagine a line falling from your shoulder, and stand so that it falls just forward of your ankle.
2. Keep your knees flexed.
3. Keep your shoulders back. You don't have to stand at attention, but you should be close to it.
4. Hold your abdomen in. Even if you're not overweight, poor posture can give you a protruding abdomen.
5. Hold your head high. This gives you the appearance of confidence and reduces aching shoulders as well.

Benefits of Good Posture

Here are some advantages of good posture:

1. It gives a feeling of confidence.
2. Good posture helps build good health by allowing the inner organs room to function properly.
3. Standing up straight helps improve your speech by freeing the power source of your voice; the diaphragm.
4. Proper body alignment contributes to a dynamic personality.

Correct Sitting Posture

There is a correct posture for sitting as well as standing. Correct sitting posture is described as follows:

1. Place your feet on the floor directly under your knees.
2. Adjust the seat of the chair to be even with your knees. This will cause the upper and lower legs to form a 90⁰ angle at the knees.
3. Allow your feet to carry the weight of your thighs.
4. Rest the weight of your torso on the thigh bones, not on the end of your spine.
5. Keep your torso erect.
6. Make sure your chair is at the correct height, so that the upper and lower parts of your arm form a right angle when you are working.

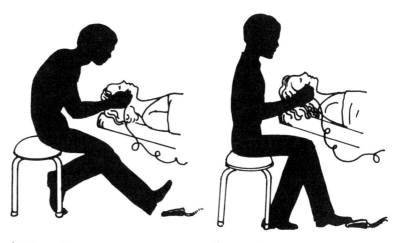

Incorrect   Correct

The correct sitting position is important because it will help you avoid general fatigue and back strain. Sit with the lower back against the chair, leaning slightly forward while servicing the client. If a stool is used, sit on the entire stool. Keep your chest up. Rest your body weight upon the full length of your thighs. To avoid back strain while reading, writing, or studying, sit well back in the chair. Do not sit in a slouching position at any time.

Correct Lifting Technique

When you lift something heavy, be sure to use the weight lifters' method or you may cause a rupture or a slipped disk. Lift with your back straight and your knees bent, pushing with the heavy thigh muscles, never with the back muscles. Also, know the weight of the object you are about to lift. You can hurt your back just as severely by lifting a light object your muscles expected to be heavy as you can by lifting a heavy object incorrectly.

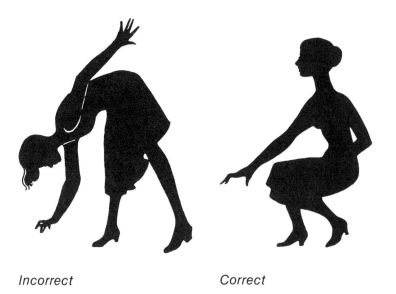

Incorrect   *Correct*

To pick up an article from the floor:

1. Place your feet close together.
2. Keep your back perpendicular to the floor as you bend your knees.
3. Lift with the muscles of your legs and buttocks, not with the back.

GROOMING THE HANDS AND FEET

It is important for the electrologist to pay special attention to the grooming of the hands and feet. A patient will rarely expect perfection on the part of the electrologist, but there is no excuse for the electrologist to have bitten nails, ragged cuticles, and rough, red hands.

Suggestions For Hand Care

1. When you must place your hands in a harsh solution, wear plastic or rubber gloves.
2. Use a protective hand cream or lotion after washing your hands and at bedtime.
3. Keep the cuticles pushed back. Use a cream or oil to keep cuticles soft. Push back the cuticles with a soft cloth after washing your hands.
4. Nail polish, colored or clear, should never be smeared or chipped. Apply fresh polish as often as needed.
5. Nails should not be too long and should never be pointed. Nails that are too long can interfere with your work or scratch a patient.
6. If you bite or pick your nails, you must break this habit. Ragged, bitten nails are unsightly, and your bad habit will be noticed by your patients.

Care of Feet

Poorly fitted shoes are often responsible for poor posture, malformed feet, and aching backs. Women should avoid extremely high heels because they throw the weight of the body forward, placing an extra strain on the feet and back.

Well-fitted shoes give the body support and balance for good posture. Wearing the correct shoes contributes to greater comfort and tends to offset the fatigue of prolonged standing. Keep toenails filed smooth. Corns, bunions, or ingrown nails should receive care from a podiatrist.

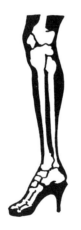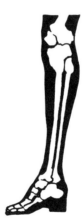

Shoes with extremely high heels will contribute to incorrect body alignment and fatigue.

Sensible shoes that support the arch will help prevent fatigue.

Giving the feet a few minutes daily care is essential to good posture and good health. You'll feel and act a lot more pleasant if your feet feel good!

Normal and Weak Arches

A normal footprint is narrow at the middle and wider at the heel and toes. Good arches are characteristic of the normal footprint.

A weak footprint is caused by a weak arch. Its footprint is wider in the middle than a normal footprint.

Fallen arches or flat feet are a common foot ailment. The flat foot leaves a footprint that is almost the same width throughout its entire length.

Weak or flat feet may be eased by means of massage, exercise, or arch supports and proper shoes. These remedial measures should be taken only after consultation with a foot specialist.

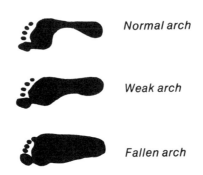

Normal arch

Weak arch

Fallen arch

QUESTIONS FOR REVIEW:

1. What are the areas of healthful living related to personal and public hygiene?
2. What are the benefits of regular exercise?
3. Why is a healthy attitude important?
4. What are the rules to follow for personal cleanliness and good health?
5. Why is good posture important?
6. What are the rules for good posture?
7. How should you care for hands and feet?

Chapter 19 Your Personality and Human Relations

LEARNING OBJECTIVES

Successful mastery of the material in this chapter will be indicated when you can:

1. List desirable qualities to cultivate.
2. Discuss the importance of voice tones and conversational skills.
3. Relate the projection of a professional personality to success as an electrologist.

INTRODUCTION

Your personality is the key to a successful career. Only you can draft the pattern of the "you" which will be most helpful in the business world. Without a pleasing personality, excellent skills or an attractive appearance will be overlooked.

DESIRABLE QUALITIES TO CULTIVATE
Attitude and Self-Discipline

Attitude has a great deal to do with personality. It influences your likes and dislikes as well as your response to people, events and things. Healthy people meet difficult situations with calmness and are cheerful, pleasant, and easy to get along with.

Control Your Temper

Control your temper. Once you have spoken, you cannot take back a single word. One person with a bad temper can throw others into a state of confusion. Everything you say or do starts a chain of reactions which, be they good or bad, will have a continuing and lasting effect. True mastery of your behavior will allow you to cultivate those characteristics which are desirable and to discard those which are unwanted.

Emotional Stability

Emotional Stability—Practice self-control. Realize that serenity is a great asset and strive for emotional balance. If you want to be successful as an electrologist, develop the qualities that command respect. Chief among these is emotional stability. Learn to suppress signs that betray negative emotions, such as facial grimaces or gestures betraying anger, impatience, envy, or greed.

Graciousness

Amiability—Learn to display positive emotions. A smile of greeting and a word of welcome, the willingness to assume the responsibilities of friendship, the ability to fit into new situations and to meet new people with friendliness, all are parts of professionalism. A sincere smile sets the mood for warm human relations.

Politeness

Politeness—The root of politeness is thoughtfulness of others. The polite professional makes "thank you," and "please," a permanent part of his or her vocabulary. He or she treats people with respect, exercises care with other people's property, is tolerant and understanding of other people's efforts, and is considerate of his or her co-workers.

Sense of Humor

Sense of Humor—Cultivate your sense of humor. Take yourself less seriously. When you can laugh at yourself, you have gained the ability to evaluate your relative personal importance.

Remember, a pleasant personality is the key to success. Be sure to develop yours to the utmost.

VOICE AND CONVERSATION

Voice and conversation, plus proper English, equal success. The use of correct English paired with intelligent conversation will prove advantageous to the professional electrologist.

Success is not made in the office alone, but depends also on personal contacts, associations, and active participation in many social and business functions.

A pleasant voice will give your words a friendly tone. Your voice should be properly pitched to further the positive effect. A monotonous voice is dull and uninteresting.

The necessity of using proper English, cultivating a pleasant voice, and developing an interesting conversational manner is not limited to contact with patients. To make progress within the profession, these essentials must be relied upon during association meetings, conventions, workshops, and social gatherings where you will come in contact with the people who create, develop, and direct electrology activities.

Your Voice is You

A satisfactory speaking voice should complement the physical self. You cannot separate what you say from what you are. The voice should convey:

1. Sincerity—honesty of mind or intention.
2. Intelligence—the ability to understand.
3. Friendliness—amiable behavior.
4. Vitality—vigor and liveliness.
5. Flexibility—the use of pliable, not rigid voice tones.
6. Expressiveness—the demonstration of one's individuality.

Tone of Voice

The tone of voice is a living expression of personality and individual effectiveness. It betrays many emotions including anger, joy, hate, love, jealousy, friendliness, and envy.

The voice should be clear and understandable, and should use adequate volume without being harsh. If the spoken words cannot be understood, a good voice tone is useless.

To be successful, a pleasing voice is needed:

1. To greet the patient.
2. For professional and social conversation.
3. To sell yourself.

4. To sell services and products.
5. To help build business.
6. To talk on the telephone.

Conversation

Conversation includes the use of voice, speech, intelligence, and personality.

The use of good speech is vital to the art of conversation. The most serious violations of good English are the use of slang, vulgarism, and poor grammar.

Topics of conversation should be as noncontroversial as possible. Friendly relations are easily achieved through pleasant conversation.

Topics to Discuss

The following topics can be discussed without controversy:

1. The patient's interests
2. The patient's activities
3. Fashion
4. Literature
5. Art
6. Music
7. Education
8. Travel
9. Civic affairs
10. Vacations

Try to understand the patient's state of mind and fit your conversation to the patient's mood, temperament, and interests.

Conversational Ease

To acquire conversational ease:

1. Guide the conversation.
2. Do not be argumentative.
3. Be a good listener.
4. Do not monopolize the conversation.
5. Do not become personal by prying into private affairs.
6. Talk about ideas rather than about specific people.
7. Use simple, easily understood language.
8. Never gossip. (Gossip is small talk used by uninteresting people.)
9. Be pleasant.
10. Use proper English.

Topics to Avoid

Never discuss the following topics:

1. Your own personal problems.
2. Religion.
3. Other patient's poor behavior.
4. Your electrology colleagues in a negative manner.
5. Your personal affairs.
6. Your own financial status.
7. Poor workmanship of co-workers.
8. Your own health problems.
9. Information given you in confidence.

Traits to Avoid

Unpopular people annoy or irritate others. To become popular, develop a desirable personality by adhering to the following rules:

1. Don't intimidate others by acting superior.
2. Avoid sarcastic remarks.
3. Never ridicule people.
4. Control your temper.
5. Don't be rude to others.
6. Never start an argument.
7. Do not talk continually about yourself.
8. Never spread gossip about anyone.
9. Avoid the use of profanity, slang, or poor grammar.
10. Don't monopolize the conversation.

NOTE: *Make a list of other rules for the professional electrologist.*

PROFESSIONAL PROJECTION

In addition to being well-groomed and proficient in your work, learning to do the little things that will make clients like you will ensure success. The professional electrologist must realize that the client's first impression of the office and its staff will often be a lasting impression. Nothing can make up for a bad first impression. For this reason, everything in the office should be in readiness before the patient arrives, with the electrologist standing by to perform the service that has been requested. A good first impression of the office and its employees will make it easier for the patient to accept any unexpected problems that may be encountered.

Every Patient is a V.I.P.

Every patient should be treated as a "very important person." No difference in attitude should be shown, nor should less service be given to a person who is less famous or less important than another. The following rules will help:

1. Always project sincerity, tact, and diplomacy.
2. Be alert, cheerful, and enthusiastic. Your attitude can make the difference as to whether or not the patient will be back.
3. Practice patience and courtesy, and show that you have a sense of humor even when things go wrong.
4. Cultivate the habits of orderliness and punctuality.
5. Practice good posture and present yourself in a professional manner at all times.
6. Be honest, dependable, and loyal.
7. Use correct grammar and speak in a pleasant manner when you talk with people, either in person or by telephone.
8. Avoid procrastination and the waste of valuable time.
9. Avoid arguments and excuses. Don't gossip.
10. Take the initiative to get work done efficiently.
11. Be helpful to co-workers, and show your employer that you are concerned with the success of the business.
12. Constantly find ways to improve yourself in your personal life and in your career.

QUESTIONS FOR REVIEW:

1. What are desirable qualities to cultivate?
2. What is the importance of voice tone and conversational skills to success as an electrologist?
3. How will projecting a professional personality aid in your success as an electrologist?

Chapter 20 The Consultation

LEARNING OBJECTIVES

Successful mastery of the material in this chapter will be indicated when you can:

1. Explain how the professional electrologist should handle a telephone consultation.
2. Describe the atmosphere for a successful silent consultation.
3. Explain the electrologist's role during the verbal consultation.
4. Define constant consultation, and explain why it is necessary.
5. Answer at least five questions the patient is likely to ask.

INTRODUCTION

As you pursue your education and training, take special care to develop your communication skills. As a successfull electrologist, you will value these skills when dealing with your patients. Good consultation techniques are essential for a successful practice.

It is important that the patient understands the treatment; how it works, how long it takes, how it heals, and whether or not hair will "regrow."

Patients must understand what electrology involves. They must be given an explanation of the technique used and given an estimate of the amount of time needed for successful treatment. These questions must be answered honestly and simply. This is because the patient has not studied electrology, and could be frightened by an excess of technical information.

Four distinct phases of consultation will be discussed.

1. Telephone consultation
2. "Silent consultation"
3. Verbal consultation
4. Constant consultation

TELEPHONE CONSULTATION

The first contact with a patient is nearly always by telephone. Remember that first impressions are very important. The caller wants to hear a confident, knowledgeable professional answer their questions.

Most often they will ask, "What does it cost?" "How long does it take?" "Does it hurt?," or even, "Does it scar?" The electrologist should listen carefully to the caller, try to calm any fears, but postpone answering these questions over the phone.

As in any professional service, the best way to answer these questions properly is with a personal consultation. When the patient is in your office, you can see the problem, explain your procedures, and estimate time and cost. Each case must be determined individually according to the sensitivity of the patient, the skin type, and the type and quantity of hair to be removed. Therefore, it is best to convince the caller to come to your office for a free consultation.

The telephone consultation should be short, honest, and polite. Remember that is only the first step to a good office consultation.

"SILENT CONSULTATION"

The nervous newcomer who steps into your office should immediately see its professional atmosphere. The reception area should be clean, well decorated, and have framed diplomas or certificates indicating your education and licensure *(LEYE sen shur)*. Articles about electrology treatment and yourself are also advantageous. Soft, pleasant music will soothe the visitor and help ease nervousness. Keep the office fragrant to please the patient's sense of smell, but make sure that the scent is not overpowering.

All of this will show concern for the patient. He or she will appreciate your concern and will respect your professional attitude.

VERBAL CONSULTATION

The verbal consultation begins when you introduce yourself. This is a critical moment for your potential patient.

Compliment the visitor's clothes or general appearance to help make the mood positive and relaxed. The person's tensions will be lessened and they will feel better. Once again they will have a good impression of you. Be careful not to patronize, however or you will have the opposite effect.

The time you spend on the verbal consultation will depend upon your experience and the patient's particular case. After several of these consultations with different patients, you will develop a pattern or formula that will give you all the facts in a minimum amount of time.

Use brochures and pamphlets that answer most commonly asked questions. These brochures can be obtained from professional associations and should be available in the reception area, and will back up your consultation and explanations. Before-and-after photographs are also an excellent tool.

It must always be explained that electrology takes time. With experience, you should be able to give the patient an approximation of the time and cost required to treat each particular problem. Case history cards will help you document your treatments, and can be used as a reference for future appointments.

It is important to explain that once an area is cleared, a few hairs may grow from untreated follicles and follow-up treatments will be necessary. Once all the hair follicles are destroyed, however, no further growth will be possible.

**CONSTANT
CONSULTATION**

Each patient visit begins another phase of your constant consultation. The consultation never ends. Use patience to repeat and explain the information over and over again until the patient understands completely what it is you are doing.

Once he or she understands, you can proceed with treatment and even continue into other areas as requested. This is one of the first indications of successful consultation, the second being the patient's delight with your services.

Once you feel you have given your new patient enough information and have obtained their confidence, you may proceed to give a short treatment (never give an extended treatment to a new patient on the first visit, especially if they've never had treatment before). This will reassure the patient and will enable you, the practitioner, to evaluate the sensitivity of the skin to determine the amount of time you will book for future visits.

**MOST FREQUENTLY
ASKED QUESTIONS**

The electrology patient will ask many questions about the anticipated procedure. The electrologist will show professional confidence and expertise by answering each one.

**Does Electrology Always
Work?**

This question is usually asked when patients see hair appearing in the treated area. Hair that appears in the area is not necessarily hair growing from a treated follicle. Most, in fact, will grow from untreated follicles. If the hair appears in six weeks or less, you can be sure that it is from a follicle that was previously dormant. Seven to eight weeks would be required for a hair to grow from the treated follicle.

**Can Electrology Be
Harmful or Cause
Scarring?**

Under normal conditions, there are no harmful effects from electrology treatment. Most undesirable aftereffects are caused by the patient. Scratching, picking, or using heavy makeup, and of course general uncleanliness, can cause problems. Caution should be taken with diabetics *(deye a BET iks)* and patients prone to keloids *(KEE loids)*. To avoid harming the patient, *the electrologist should not treat areas inside the nose or ears, or wherever there are skin irritations,* until the patient has been examined by a physician.

**Can Hair Be Removed
From a Mole?**

The electrologist should check insurance coverage and state regulations before treating a mole. A physician's permission should also be obtained to protect the health of the patient. These precautions are presently necessary because treating moles is still controversial. There is no recorded damage due to treatment of a mole, and many insurance companies now cover this treatment.

**How Long Does Each
Treatment Last?**

The average treatment ranges from 15 minutes to one hour. The amount of time per treatment depends upon the reaction of the skin to treatment, and the patient's sensitivity. Timing also depends on what part of the body is being treated. The first treatment should last no more than 15 minutes. Use this treatment as a test. If all goes well, a patient may eventually receive three hours of body treatment at one time. Facial treatments will always vary greatly depending upon the area; from 15 minutes to one hour.

How Much Hair Can Be Removed in One Treatment?

The amount of hair that can be removed in one treatment depends upon the sensitivity of the patient, the skin, and the proficiency of the electrologist.

Can I Get an Infection From the Treatment?

Infection can result from electrology treatment, although it is rare. Infections are most commonly caused by the patient after treatment, and are usually of a minor cosmetic nature. This type of infection will clear within 3 to 8 weeks. *It is crucial that the electrologist use sterilization (ster i li ZAY shun) and sanitation, (san i TAY shun) procedures to decrease the possibility of infection.*

Why Does Hair Regrow?

There are many reasons for hair regrowth. Sometimes an insertion is not accurate and misses the dermal papilla, resulting in regrowth.

If the insertion is accurate, but only destroys the dermal papilla and not the lower two-thirds of the hair follicle where the germinative cells are located, hair will regrow.

A hair treated in the telogen, or resting stage, will probably not be affected by electrology treatment.

Will Hyperpigmentation Always Occur After Treatment?

Not always. Hyperpigmentation *(HEYE per PIG men TAY shun)* or freckling of the treated area, is possible, especially if the hair is dark, deep, terminal hair. Most cases of hyperpigmentation clear within a few months, but in some cases it can last for as long as 24 months.

Will Electrology Treatment Stimulate New Hair Growth?

Some experts feel that the stimulation can cause a few surrounding follicles to grow hair. This has not been scientifically proven.

Is One Electrology Method Most Effective?

There are three acceptable modalities for permanent hair removal at the present time. The efficiency of the method depends totally on the practitioner, not the equipment.

What Is the Black Material that Appears on the Skin After Treatment?

It can be identified as the remnants of a club hair. This occurs when a hair is treated in the later stages of telogen with an early anagen hair already growing beneath it. If both hairs are successfully treated, the anagen hair will appear at the skin surface days later.

There is also the possibility of hair breakage during removal. This will leave the thick root portion in the follicle. It will appear on the surface a few days to a week after treatment.

What Is the White Tissue that Appears Soon After Treatment?

The white tissue is the sheath *(sheeth)*, or the covering around the hair itself. As the hair is removed from the follicle, the sheath will occasionally peel off.

Does Temporary Hair Removal Affect Hair Growth?

Stimulation of the dermal papilla can cause hair to grow wider in diameter, and at times can distort the hair follicle. Only tweezing or waxing can cause enough trauma to stimulate the dermal papilla. Cutting, shaving, and depilatories do not reach the dermal papilla and do not affect growth.

A patient under treatment should not tweeze between sessions, but may cut any visible hairs until their next appointment.

Patients who have distorted hairs due to temporary removal methods should be advised to space appointments closely so that you can treat hairs in their early anagen phase. At that point the hair is straight and the papilla is closer to the surface of the skin, making electrology more effective.

Why Does the Skin Scab After Treatment?

Electrology causes microscopic hemorrhaging, so it is normal for scabs to form after treatment, especially on the lower areas of the body. The patient must be advised not to pick scabs or they will leave small pits.

What Causes Ingrown Hairs?

Ingrown hairs grow through the side of the follicle and lie just beneath the skin's surface. Ingrown hairs are usually caused by tweezing or waxing, when the hair breaks at the weakest point just below the surface of the skin. This can distort the hair, especially if it is pulled against its direction of growth. The hair will then grow under the surface of the skin rather than up and out of the hair follicle. A pimple-like inflammation results that is uncomfortable to the patient, especially when it occurs on the inner thigh, the neck, or the underarm.

Men with heavy beards can have this problem. When they shave close, the hair pulls back into the hair follicle, and sometimes its direction of growth is altered, causing ingrown hairs.

Patients who are prone to ingrown hairs should stop tweezing or waxing and receive electrology treatments immediately.

Does Electrology Treatment Hurt?

The sensation is less than in tweezing. Most patients are suprised as they expect to feel much more. Some patients even relax enough to fall asleep.

What Areas of the Body Are Most Sensitive?

The upper lip and the inner thighs are the most sensitive areas.

Can the Breast Be Treated During Pregnancy?

Medical authorities feel there is no problem. It is best to leave this decision to the patient, however, as some women are more sensitive during pregnancy.

Can a Local Anesthesia Be Given?

Yes, but only by a qualified dentist or physician. Many patients may want this, particularly for the upper lip or inner thigh. The electrologist must be extremely careful not to overtreat these areas.

Will the Pore Be Larger After Treatment?

The size of the pore is due to the size of the hair treated. The electrologist must make the patient aware of this before treatment, as pores are more evident once the hair is removed.

Can Children Be Treated?

Unless prohibited by state regulations, children may be treated. It is, of course, wise to have the permission of the parents of children under legal age. You may occasionally be asked to treat a child against his or her wishes. If at all possible, avoid the treatment.

CONCLUSION

One last note. You may become the finest practitioner in the world, giving first class consultations and services, and still have a patient stop treatment. Any service that treats the public is complex. Many factors of which you are unaware are involved, such as personality, and personal and financial pressures. Always give your very best and don't be upset if a patient chooses to discontinue.

Another important consideration is for your colleagues. In any consultation and resulting treatment, remember to speak of your competition only in a positive manner. This is professional and ethical conduct. Remember this regardless of the patient's legitimate cause to complain.

Electrology is a profession as well as a business. It's a profession which helps make people happier about themselves. To be a part of the profession you must always have an honest concern for the patient. This, above all, must be conveyed in the four phases of consultation.

QUESTIONS FOR REVIEW:

1. How should the professional electrologist handle the telephone consultation?
2. What should the atmosphere in the professional electrologist's office be like? Why should it be that way?
3. How should the electrologist act during the verbal consultation?
4. What is the meaning of constant consultation? Why is it necessary?
5. What are five questions the patient is likely to ask? How should you answer?

Chapter 21 Starting an Electrology Practice

LEARNING OBJECTIVES Successful mastery of the material in this chapter will be indicated when you can:

1. Describe possible locations to consider for an electrology practice and office.
2. Explain what insurance will cover in the electrology office.
3. Give the nine layout essentials of an electrology office.
4. List the seven advertising media options available to the electrologist.
5. List five items that contribute to good business operation.
6. Give five reasons why records are required for good business administration.
7. Describe the business law aspects of three types of ownership.

INTRODUCTION Starting your own practice is exciting, but it is also a big responsibility. It is not a step to be taken without serious planning. Knowledge of business principles, bookkeeping, business law, insurance, salesmanship, and psychology are crucial to the successful professional. Some of the advantages and disadvantages you will face in business are outlined in this chapter.

PRECONSIDERATIONS When planning to open an electrology office, give careful consideration to every aspect of running a practice. The following topics will acquaint you with some of the things you must take into account before going into business.

Location A good location will have a population large enough to support the office. When possible, the office should be located near other active businesses or a shopping center. This will help attract potential patients. People are drawn to areas where they can make one stop to accomplish several things. Unless you have a large amount of money for advertising, it is difficult to operate a successful office in a low-traffic area. An ideal location would be within a medical center that is situated near a shopping mall.

If you decide to set up your practice in your home, make sure that the office has a separate entrance and is well detached from your living quarters. This will ensure patient privacy and will give your practice a professional aspect.

The cosmetology salon is not the ideal place to begin an electrology practice, because you will usually be limited to the clientele of the salon. Many patients will not be comfortable walking through the salon to get to the electrologist's booth. They may be embarrassed or may feel the need for more privacy. This could limit your practice considerably.

Visibility

The office should be clearly visible in order to attract the attention of people walking or driving by. Professional signs in obvious locations are very effective.

Study the Area

Analyze the area for potential patients. Find out about the size, income, and buying habits of the area's population. Talk to other business owners and professionals to see how they feel an electrology office would be accepted. Talk to local dermatologists, physicians, and cosmetologists to get their input regarding potential patients. This will also help you to determine a proper fee.

Study Lease

Always negotiate leases and work arrangements legally, and be sure you understand all lease restrictions for your landlord as well as yourself. The lease should provide for alterations that must be made. It is advisable to have a lawyer help you with negotiations before you sign a lease. A sink and toilet facilities are essential.

Parking Facilities

When selecting a site for a new practice or planning to take over an established practice, you must consider parking. People hesitate to patronize an office which has inadequate parking space. Make sure there is enough parking for the practice you anticipate. If your office is open for evening service, the parking area should be well lit. If possible, locate the office near a bus or train line for those patients that do not drive. A hard to reach location will deter many patients.

Written Agreements

Written agreements for labor and costs for alterations will prevent disputes over who must pay for what.

REGULATIONS, BUSINESS LAWS, AND INSURANCE

It is necessary to comply with local, state and federal regulations and laws when conducting a busines and employing help.

Regulations and Laws

Local regulations may cover building and renovations (local building codes).

Federal law covers social security and unemployment compensation or insurance.

State law covers sales taxes, licenses, and worker's compensation.

Income tax laws are covered by both state and federal governments.

Insurance covers malpractice, premises liability, fire, burglary and theft, and use of occupation policies.

**PLANNING THE
PHYSICAL LAYOUT**

The layout of the electrology office takes considerable planning in order to be efficient and economical.

**Electrology
Office**

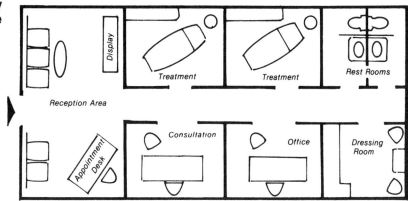

Layout Essentials

The electrology office should have:

1. Maximum efficiency of operation.
2. Flow of operational services toward the reception room.
3. Enough space for each piece of equipment.
4. Furniture, fixtures and equipment chosen on the basis of cost, durability, utility, and appearance. The purchase of standard and guaranteed equipment is a worthwhile investment.
5. A color scheme that is restful and tasteful.
6. A dispensary and plenty of storage space.
7. A clean restroom.
8. Good plumbing and sufficient lighting for satisfactory services.
9. Air conditioning and heating.
10. A covered waste container.

The reception area should not be overlooked when you plan the layout of your office. This is the first contact a patient has with your establishment and it sets the tone for the rest of the office. An attractively decorated reception area can be one of your best promotional tools. It immediately makes a patient comfortable and gives the impression that this is an office that cares about the comfort of its patients. The reception area may also be an eye-catcher for people who accompany your patients to the office. These people may become potential patients. Displaying various diplomas, before and after photos and your membership in your international electrologists organization will contribute to your credibility.

ADVERTISING

Advertising includes all activities which attract attention to the office and which create a favorable impression to the public. Your personality, ability, the quality of your treatment, and the attractiveness of your office are all natural advertising assets. By looking good yourself, you become an advertisement for your services. Always wear a white uniform or smock during office hours to project professionalism, another natural advertising asset. A satisfied patient is, of course, the best form of advertising.

Media Options

Advertising must attract and hold the person's attention and must create a desire for your services. Before starting an advertising program, be sure to plan an advertising budget.

1. Use newspaper advertising as the first medium. Local weeklies work best.
2. Use direct mail to create a more intimate contact with the reader. Mail to all physicians and salons.
3. Classified advertising in the yellow pages of your telephone book is comparatively inexpensive and extremely effective.
4. Radio advertising is more expensive, but can be very effective.
5. TV is a dramatic but expensive medium for advertising.
6. A professional window sign acts as a sales piece for every passerby.
7. Personal public appearances are excellent advertising. These may include appearances at women's and men's groups, charitable affairs, and TV talk shows.

BUSINESS OPERATION AND PERSONNEL MANAGEMENT

When starting a business, it is very important to know what your **overhead** is. Overhead is simply your total business expenses. The majority of electrologists go out of business because they do not have a clear picture of what their expenses and rent will be before they open their practice.

Causes of Failure

Some of the most common causes of failure are:

1. Inexperience in dealing with the public and with employees.
2. Not enough capital to carry the business through until it is established, poor location, and excessively high overhead expenses.
3. Lack of proper basic training in the field.
4. Business neglect and careless bookkeeping.

Ways To Success

The owner of an electrology office must have business sense, knowledge, ability, good judgment, and diplomacy. Smooth management depends upon:

1. Sufficient investment capital.
2. Efficiency of management.
3. Cooperation between management, employees and patients.
4. Good business procedures.
5. Trained and experienced personnel in the office.

Allocation of Money
As part of your business operation, you must always know where your money is being spent. It is always a good idea to budget your money so that maximum benefit is obtained.

Make a list of your average expenses:

AVERAGE EXPENSES

(Based on total gross income)

	Percent
Salaries and commissions (including payroll taxes)	*53.5*
Rent	*13*
Supplies	*5*
Advertising	*3*
Depreciation	*3*
Laundry	*1*
Cleaning	*1*
Light and power	*1*
Repairs	*1.5*
Insurance	*.75*
Telephone	*.75*
Miscellaneous expenses	*1.5*
Total expense	*85*
Net profit	*15*

You will note that the largest items of expense are rent, advertising, and supplies. These items, then, need your closest attention. You can adjust advertising as needed.

When opening an electrology office, it is important to have enough working capital. It takes time to build a new practice, so money must be available to take care of necesary expenses. As overhead is met and profits increase, the budget can be adjusted to cover more advertising and to expand in other areas.

Booking Appointments
Book appointments with care, for this can make the difference between success and failure. services are sold in terms of time on the appointment page. That time, depending on how it is used, may spell either gain or loss. The "Week at a Glance" appointment book is an effective instrument for organizing your time. Be certain to stay within the time frame for each client, and to allow sufficient time for the services requested.

BUSINESS ADMINISTRATION
Good business administration demands keeping a simple and efficient record system. Records are valuable only if they are correct, concise, and complete. Bookkeeping means maintaining accurate records of all income and expenses. Income is money received for services and from retail sales. Expenses include rent, utilities, insurance, salaries, advertising, equipment, and repairs. It may be valuable to hire an accountant to help you with these records. Keep check stubs, cancelled checks, receipts, and invoices.

You will need to keep business records in order to meet the requirements of local, state, and federal laws regarding taxes and employees.

Reasons for Proper Records

All business transactions must be recorded in order to maintain proper records, which are required of the owner of an electrology office for the following reasons:

1. Efficient operation of the office.
2. Determining income, expenses, profit, and loss.
3. Proving the value of the office to prospective buyers.
4. Arranging bank loans.
5. Reports of income tax, social security, unemployment and disability insurance, wage and hour law, accident compensation, and labor tax.

Daily Records

Keeping daily records allows you to know just how the practice is progressing. Make sure you keep a record of every patient that comes into your office so you will know their case history. Furthermore, a weekly or monthly summary will help to:

1. Make comparisons with other years.
2. Order necessary supplies.
3. Control expenses and waste.

Each expense item affects the total gross income. Accurate records will show the cost of your operation in relation to its income.

Keep a daily income record, appointment book, and petty cash book. The payroll book, cancelled checks, and monthly and yearly records are usually held for at least seven years. Service and inventory records are also important in that they will enable you to avoid running short of supplies needed for services. They will also help you establish net worth at the end of the year.

BUSINESS LAW FOR THE OFFICE

An office may be owned and operated by an individual, a partnership, or a corporation. Before you decide which type of ownership is best, you should be acquainted with the relative merits of each.

Individual Ownership

The aspects of individual ownership are as follows:

1. You are boss and manager.
2. You can determine policies and make decisions.
3. You receive all profits and bear all losses.

Partnership

The aspects of a partnership are as follows:

1. More capital is available for investment.
2. The combined ability and experience of the partners makes it easier to share work and responsibilities, and to make decisions as well as making it easier to take needed time off.

3. Profits are equally shared.
4. Each partner assumes the other's unlimited liability for debts.

Corporation   The aspects of a corporation are as follows:

1. A charter has to be obtained from the state.
2. A corporation is subject to taxation and regulation by the state.
3. The management is in the hands of a board of directors who determine policies and make decisions in accordance with the charter.
4. Profits are divided in proportion to the number of shares held by each stockholder.
5. The stockholders are not legally responsible for losses.

Before Buying or Selling an Established Office   There are several things to keep in mind before buying or selling your practice. You should consider that:

1. A written purchase and sale agreement is necessary in order to avoid misunderstandings between the contracting parties.
2. The written agreement should be placed in the hands of an impartial third person for safekeeping and enforcement. This person is to deliver the agreement to the grantee (one to whom the property is transferred upon the fulfillment of the specified contract).
3. The buyer or seller should take and sign a complete statement of inventory (of equipment, fixtures, etc.) detailing the value of each article.
4. If there is a transfer of chattel mortgage, notes, lease and bill of sale, an investigation should be made to determine any default in the payment of debts.
5. You should consult your lawyer for additional guidance.

Agreement to Buy a Practice   An agreement to buy an established practice should include the following:

1. Correct identity of owner.
2. True representations concerning the value and inducements offered to buy the office. An up-to-date patient list should be available to you as well as past appointment books.
3. Use of office's name and reputation for a definite period of time.
4. An understanding that the seller will not compete with the prospective owner within a reasonable distance from the present location.
5. A copy of the present lease for your review.

Protection in a Lease

Protect your interests when signing a lease. The following guidelines will help:

1. Secure exemption of fixtures or appliances which may be attached to the office space, so that they can be removed without violating the lease.
2. Insert into the lease an agreement regarding necessary renovations and repairs such as painting, plumbing, fixtures, and electrical installation.
3. Secure options from the landlord to assign the lease to another person. This will keep the obligations for paying rent separate from the responsibilities of operating the business.

Protection Against Fire, Theft, and Lawsuits

It is impossible to guarantee that none of these will happen to you. The following, however, will help:

1. Employ honest and competent practitioners and keep the premises securely locked.
2. Follow safety precautions to prevent fire, injury, and lawsuits. Liability, fire, malpractice, and burglary insurance are necessary.
3. Do not violate the medical practice law of your state by attempting to diagnose, treat or cure a disease.
4. Become thoroughly familiar with all laws governing electrology, and with the sanitary codes of your city and state.
5. Keep accurate records of employees' salaries, length of employment, and social security numbers. These are needed for various state and federal laws affecting social welfare of employees.

CAUTION: *Ignorance of the law is no excuse for its violation.*

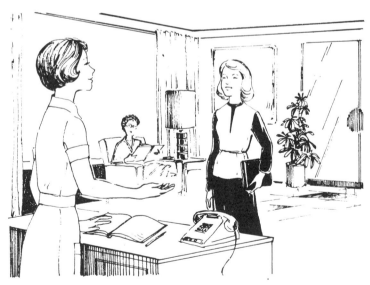

The patient's first impression of an electrology office is often a lasting one. Your office should be well-organized, attractively decorated, and should reflect a pleasant, professional atmosphere.

SUMMARY   Important things to consider when going into business:

CAPITAL
Amount available
Amount required

ORGANIZATION
Individual, partnership
corporation

BANKING
Opening a bank account
Deposits, drawing checks
Monthly statements
Notes and drafts

SELECTING LOCATION
Population
Transportation facilities
Transients
Trade possibilities
Space required
Zoning ordinances
Parking

DECORATING AND
FLOOR PLAN
Selection of furniture
Floor covering
Installing telephone
Interior decorating
Exterior decorating
Window displays
Signs

EQUIPMENT AND SUPPLIES
Selecting equipment
Comparative values
Installation
Labor-saving steps

ADVERTISING
Planning
Direct mail
Local house organs
Newspaper
Radio
Television

LEGAL
Lease, contracts
Claims and lawsuits

BOOKKEEPING SYSTEM
Installation
Record of appointments
Receipts and disbursements
Petty cash
Profit and loss
Inventory

COST OF OPERATION
Supplies, Depreciation,
Rent, Light, Salaries,
Telephone, Linen service,
Sundries, Taxes

MANAGEMENT
Methods of building goodwill
Analysis of materials and labor
 in relation to service charges
Greeting clients
Adjusting complaints
Handling employees
Selling merchandise
Telephone techniques

OFFICE ADMINISTRATION
Stationery and office supplies
Inventory

INSURANCE
Public liability and malpractice
Compensation, unemployment
Social Security
Fire, theft and burglary

METHODS OF PAYMENT
In advance
C.O.D.
Open account
Time payments

COMPLIANCE WITH
LABOR LAWS
Minimum wage law
Hours of employment
Minors

ETHICS
Courtesy
Observation of professional
 trade practices

COMPLIANCE WITH STATE LAW governing physical layout
and equipment.

LICENSING of offices and electrologists.

QUESTIONS FOR REVIEW

1. What are the possible locations for an electrology office?
2. What will insurance cover in the electrology office?
3. What are the nine layout essentials of an electrology office?
4. Which seven advertising media options are available to the electrologist?
5. What are the five things which contribute to good business operation?
6. What are the five reasons proper records are required for good business administration?
7. What are the business law aspects of three types of ownership?

Chapter 22 Psychology and Human Relations in Business

LEARNING OBJECTIVES

Successful mastery of the material in this chapter will be indicated when you can:

1. List the five principles of selling.
2. Explain how your personality relates to selling power.
3. Give at least three examples of professional sales techniques.
4. Discuss methods for building a practice.
5. Explain how your professional image is important in the employment interview.

INTRODUCTION

Sales ability is becoming an increasingly important responsibility of the electrologist. As demand for the service continues to grow and as the public increasingly views electrology as acceptable, the professional electrologist will need to sell his or her services more and more.

SALES PRINCIPLES

There are five definite principles of selling. They are:

Attention—This is the very first impression you make on the potential patient. Be certain that it is a good one by having an office that is clean and neat. Greet the person enthusiastically as they enter, and be certain that they feel comfortable.

Interest—Have before and after photographs available. Mention that you have successfully treated similar cases.

Desire—Make the person want to have electrology.

Conviction—Convince them that the services you offer will be successful, and that they will enjoy the results. Show them that electrology is the best solution to their problems.

Close—Make the appointment.

In order to accomplish all five steps successfully and have a new patient, you will need to be familiar with the merits and benefits of electrology services. You will have to be self-confident, so that you can stimulate interest and desire. It is important that you always be honest and represent your services fairly. Have several sales approaches, and be able to read human signals so that you can apply the appropriate technique. Never be negative about electrology; always show the positive results. The most important step is the close, so believe in yourself enough to ask for that appointment to begin treatment.

Types of Patients and Your Response to Them

The electrologist who is most likely to be successful in selling services to patients is the one who can recognize the many different types of people and know how to serve each type.

Here are seven basic types of people that you are likely to meet, and suggestions on how you should treat each:

1. Shy, timid—Make the shy person feel at ease. Lead the conversation. Don't force the individual to talk, but show that you care about their opinion.
2. Talkative—Be a patient listener. Tactfully switch the conversation to his or her needs.
3. Nervous, irritable—This individual does not want much conversation. Give good, efficient service with a pleasant smile.
4. Inquisitive, over-cautious—Explain the treatment in detail.
5. Conceited, "know it all"—Be agreeable, but firm in your knowledge. Never argue. Be quick to pass a compliment.
6. Young (teenage)—Don't oversell. Give special advice for aftercare.
7. Mature—Be courteous and solicitous of mature patients. Suggest services suitable for mature persons.

PERSONALITY AND SELLING POWER

Your selling power will increase progressively as you make patients aware of your personal interest in their welfare. Treat all patients with friendliness and extend courtesies with a warm greeting and a pleasant smile.

Positive Qualities

The following are some positive qualities necessary for a successful career:

Optimism—the expectation that things will come out all right.

Acquisitiveness—the desire to acquire wealth and improve your position in life.

Self assertiveness—the ability to realize that a problem is an opportunity.

Initiative—the ability to do what is necessary without being told what to do or how to do it.

Cheerfulness—a congenial spirit which makes the work of selling services pleasant for you and your patient.

Tact—saying or doing the right thing at the right time, in the right place.

Sincerity—making your suggestions because you really believe the treatment will be a good one for the patient.

Ability to smile—a smiling face tells the patient that you are pleased to provide service.

Good image—look, act, speak, and know the part of the professional electrologist.

Sales Psychology

No matter how good a service may be, you will find it difficult to make a sale, unless there is a need for it. Before attempting to sell a treatment, first determine whether the patient really needs it. Every person who enters your office is an individual. Determine what that patient needs before you attempt to sell it.

What are the motives which prompt people to desire electrology? People want to make the most of their good features and to hide their bad features. Personal satisfaction will make them buy from you. Find their strongest desire, center your appeal around it, and you will sell your services.

If a patient is doubtful or undecided, help them make the decision by giving honest and sincere advice. Show that patient what the treatment involves, and how it will provide a benefit.

PROFESSIONAL SALES TECHNIQUES

The best interests of the patient should be your first consideration. Under no circumstances should you approach a patient only with the thought of the amount of money you can get. Sincerity, honesty, and good service pay off in a loyal patient list.

Carefully consider each patient's needs. Use tact and diplomacy as well as courtesy if you want the patient's continued patronage.

Describe the Benefits of Service

Each service requires the correct sales technique, using simple and suggestive language which will make the patient feel like buying. Create interest and desire by using picture words, descriptive adjectives, and feeling. Present the patient with a verbal picture of the benefits of electrology treatments.

Personalize Your Selling

Learn to identify patients not only by appearance, but also by name. Address a patient by his or her last name until you are asked to use the first name. Keep a record card indicating skin type, nature of treatment, and the fee. When the patient calls again, you can refresh your memory regarding the last appointment. Record cards also tell your patient that you have a personal interest in them.

Every client is a potential source of new patients. A satisfied individual will boost the reputation of the electrologist and, as a result, will bring in new patients. Encourage the patient to take a series of treatments so that they may see the desired result quickly and effectively.

When selling office treatments, stress quality and permanence over cheaper alternatives. You might say, "Although it seems like you are paying more, electrolysis is actually less expensive than a lifetime of shaving, waxing or using depilatory creams.

BUILDING A PRACTICE   Loyal patients are a steady source of income. For this reason it is wise to take the time to build a practice; to become known. Patients who like your work will come back again and they will ask for you. They will also recommend you and the office to their friends and associates. Successful electrologists can look back and remember when they started with only a few patients. When they were not busy providing a service, however, they were not idle. They always found something to do or someone from whom they could learn. An electrologist can be helpful to others by taking case histories, or can help in other ways. The practitioner has to build the image of him or herself as one who specializes in the field of electrology.

Publicity   There are many ways to get free publicity. Many clubs and organizations are interested in having speakers who can entertain their group and possibly demonstrate a service. This is a good way to advertise your work and your place of business, and will often be written up for the local press.

You will be required to speak on electrology and possibly demonstrate the techniques involved. This will give you the opportunity to speak with students and parents who may be interested in treatment. You will be helping students who may want to go into the field, and you may even get coverage by local media if you plan carefully. Joining your state or national electrolysis association could be a great opportunity to learn about the promotion through public relations. Look around for other opportunities for free publicity. Advertising in your local yellow pages, weekly newspapers, direct mail announcements, and contacting your neighborhood physicians are usually your best forms of publicity.

YOUR PROFESSIONAL IMAGE AND THE EMPLOYMENT INTERVIEW   Over the years, many dedicated people have worked hard to build the image of the field of electrology. As a student you are also building your personal image and contributing to the image the public has of your profession. Professional pride, professional knowledge, and the projection of a professional attitude all start in the classroom as part of your preparation for a career. Once you have passed the necessary tests and have qualified, you are ready to put your knowledge and skills to work as a professional electrologist. It will be to your advantage if you begin researching the jobs and opportunities that are available before you graduate. There is no magic formula that makes job hunting easy, but your attitude can help. If you feel ill at ease and apprehensive, study the following suggestions and give yourself a personal evaluation. Work on the areas where you need improvement and compliment yourself on your many good qualities.

Personal Evaluation   1. Employers in service careers place special emphasis on a healthy, well-groomed appearance, so be sure you plan your appearance carefully for the employment interview. When in doubt about what to wear, be conservative. This doesn't mean that you have to look drab, but wear what is most appropriate for the professional image you wish to project. In some cases it may be appropriate to wear a uniform, but you will not normally be expected to wear it for the employment interview. Makeup should be discreet and hair must be clean and neat and styled attractively. Nails should be manicured. Beards and mustaches should be neatly trimmed, or the face freshly shaven.

2. Don't smoke or chew gum during your interview. Either will detract from your professionalism.

3. Project confidence through your posture while sitting and standing. A slouching posture will make you appear insecure and uninterested.

4. Try to anticipate the questions you may be asked at the interview so you can be prepared. The main purpose of the employment interview is to match the place of business to the best person for the job. The person conducting the interview will usually take the lead in conversation and will put you at ease. He or she will explain company policy, salary, commission, benefits, working hours, and other important information. If this information is not given, you may tactfully ask what is offered.

When you go for the interview, keep in mind that you have knowledge and skills to offer. You will not be expected to take a job without first knowing what wages you will receive and what will be expected of you. You are looking for an opportunity to build a satisfying career, and the employer is looking for someone who can contribute to the growth and financial success of the place of business. It will be to your advantage to start in a practice that offers you the best opportunities to learn and grow in your profession.

The Resume The resume will often not be required when you apply for a job, but it is a good idea to have one prepared. It will provide you with information for filling out application forms, and will project an image of professionalism. You should anticipate being asked to demonstrate your practical skills.

How to Find Leads for Job Opportunities You will be ahead of the game if you start looking into possible job opportunities before you graduate. Your school counselor will usually be able to assist you and keep you informed of opportunities. Offices will often work with a school to find new staff. In addition, you may wish to do the following:

1. Watch the daily newspapers and association newsletters for leads such as announcements for the opening of new offices or practices for sale. Check the help wanted ads to see if your qualifications match those needed for the jobs advertised.

2. Check advertisements in trade journals, professional magazines, and other publications. If you apply by letter, be sure to enclose a resume and ask for a personal interview.

3. Check with your family, friends, neighbors, teachers or anyone who may know of someone looking for an employee with your qualifications.

4. Look in the classified section of your telephone directory for names of firms or offices which interest you, and then apply to them directly. You may wish to call to see if they will give you a personal interview.

5. Find out what beginners in your field can expect to be paid so that you will be able to discuss salary intelligently during the interview. You must consider transportation to and from your job and the amount of money you will need to live. Sometimes a job may pay less to start, but will offer opportunities for growth and other benefits you will want to consider.

6. Be adaptable in terms of the hours you are willing to work and the location in which you will work. You may have a better opportunity if you work evenings, weekends, or a split shift, and you may have less competition in outlying areas.

7. Be prepared in the following ways: Be able to tell the interviewer why you would like to work for him or her. Have your social security card and certificate or license with you. Have a resume with accurate information about yourself. Include information about your education and the dates you attended school. List experience related to the job you are seeking. Also list the names, addresses, and telephone numbers of people you have as references.

8. Be optimistic. If you are asked to fill out forms or take tests, do so cheerfully. Don't be discouraged if you don't do as well as you thought you might. If you don't get this job, keep trying because some other job may be better for you.

9. If you really want the job you have been interviewed for, it is courteous and often helpful to write a short note to thank the interviewer.

10. Don't forget to find out all you can about the business before the interview. Since you will be spending a lot of time on the job, it is better to know any negative aspects of the job before you are hired. If for some reason you do make a mistake and find yourself in the wrong job, remember that nothing learned is ever lost. Practice your professional ethics when giving notice that you are leaving a job and always leave with goodwill.

QUESTIONS FOR REVIEW:

1. What sales principles are necessary?
2. How does your personality relate to selling power?
3. What are three examples of professional sales techniques?
4. How can you build a practice?
5. How is your professional image important during the employment interview?

Electrology Glossary

A

abdominal *(ab DOM i nahl)*: relating to the area of the body below the chest and diaphram; contains digestive organs.

abnormal *(ab NOR mahl)*: irregular; contrary to the natural law or customary order.

absorption *(ab SORP shun)*: the assimilation of one body through another; act of absorbing.

acanthosis *(ak an THOH sis)*: a condition that is the result of an increased number of prickle cells.

Achard Thiers Syndrome *(ash AHR TEERZ SIN drohm)*: diabetes and hirsutism in post menopausal women.

acid *(AH sid)*: any of a class of substances containing hydrogen that can be replaced by a metal to form a salt.

acidity *(ah SID i tee)*: being acid.

acne *(AK nee)*: a chronic inflammatory disorder of the skin, usually related to hormonal changes and overactive sebaceous glands during adolescence, (also known as acne simplex or acne vulgaris).

acne vulgaris *(AK nee vul GAR is)*: acne simplex; simple uncomplicated pimples.

acromegaly *(AK roh MEG ah lee)*: a condition caused by hypersecretion of the pituitary growth hormone after maturity. Largeness of skeleton, nose, jaws, fingers and toes.

actinic keratinosis *(ak TIN ik ker ah TOH NOH sis)*: a premalignant skin condition due to over-exposure to the sun.

acute *(ah CYOOT)*: means severe.

acute disease *(ah KYOOT di ZEEZ)*: is manifested by symptoms of a more or less violent character and of short duration.

adipose tissue *(AD i pohs TISH yoo)*: areolar connective tissue containing fat cells; subcutaneous tissue.

adrenal cortex *(a DREE nal KOHR teks)*: the cortical portion of the adrenal gland.

adrenal gland *(a DREE nal gland)*: an endocrine gland situated on top of the kidneys.

adrenal hyperplasia *(a DREE nal HEYE per PLAZ ee ah)*: excess growth of normal cells in the adrenal gland.

adrenal virilism *(a DREE nal VEER ah liz ahm)*: the premature development of secondary male characteristics in both male and female children (excess hair) due to a malfunction of the adrenal cortex.

adrenaline *(a DREN a lin)*: a hormone secreted by the adrenal gland; it stimulates the nervous system, raises metabolism, increases cardiac pressure and output and increases blood pressure.

adrenocorticotrophic *(ad REE noh KOHR tee koh TROF ik)*: exerting a specific effect upon the cortex of the adrenal gland.

adsorption *(ad SORP shun)*: to gather or assimilate a dissolved substance on the surface only; the skin adsorbs medicated creams.

afferent fibers *(AF er ent FEYE burs)*: the fibers that stimulate impulses to the central nervous system.

albinism *(AL bi niz em)*: congenital leucoderma or absence of pigment in the skin and its appendages; it may be partial or complete.

alcohol *(AL ko hawl)*: a readily evaporating, colorless liquid with a pungent odor and burining taste; powerful stimulant and antiseptic.

aldactone *(al DAK tohn)*: a trademark for a preparation of a diuretic agent with hydrochlorothiazide.

aldosterone *(al DOS teh ruhn)*: very important regulator of metabolism of sodium potassium.

alkalies *(AL kah leyes)*: a class of compounds which react with acids to form salts, turn red litmus paper blue, saponify fats and form soluble carbonates; having a pH number above 7.0.

alkalinity *(al hah LIN i tee)*: the quality or state of being alkaline.

allergy *(AL er gee)*: a state of hypersensitivity to certain substances.

alopecia *(AL oh PEE shee ah)*: deficiency of hair; baldness.

ampere *(AM peer)*: a measure of electrical current flow.

anabolism *(ah NAB o lizm)*: constructive metabolism; the process of assimilation of nutritive matter and its conversion into living substance.

anagen phase *(AN ah jen fayz)*: phase of hair cycle during which synthesis of hair takes place; early production phase of the hair cycle in a follicle.

anaphase *(AN ah fayz)*: the stage of mitosis and meiosis in which the chromosomes move toward the poles of the spindle.

anaphoresis *(AN ah fo REE sis)*: the process of forcing liquids into the tissues from the negative toward the positive pole. Creates lye, irritates and causes redness to the skin in small doses, can soften skin, and acts as a vaso-dilator.

anatomy *(ah NAHT o mee)*: the study of the organs and systems of the body such as muscles, bones and arteries.

androgen *(AN dro jen)*: any of various hormones that control the development of masculine characteristics; the hormone responsible for hair growth and usually the primary causes for excess hair growth when it is secreted above normal levels.

anidrosis *(an i DROH sis)*: lack of perspiration, often a result of fever or certain skin diseases. Requires medical treatment.

anorexia nervosa *(an o REK see ah nur VOH sah)*: psychological condition causing chronic absence of appetite for food has been related to excess hair growth.

anterior lobe *(an TEER i or lohb)*: portion of the pituitary gland which regulates the growth hormone.

antibiotic *(an ti beye OT ik)*: a drug, such as penicillin, made from substances derived from mold or bacterium which inhibits the growth of bacteria.

antiseptic *(an ti SEP tik):* a chemical agent that prevents the growth of bacteria.

apocrine glands *(AP o krin glands):* sweat glands that produce a distinctive odor; found in the underarms and pubic areas of the body.

arrector pili *(ah REK tor PI lee):* involuntary muscle fibers in the skin attached to the base of the hair follicles.

areola *(ah REE oh lah):* any small ring-like discoloration; the pigmented ring surrounding the nipple of the breast. Hair may surround this area and it is safely treated.

artery *(AHR te ree):* a blood vessel which conveys blood from the heart to all parts of the body.

asepsis *(ay SEP sis):* a condition in which pathogenic bacteria are present.

assimilation *(ah sim i LAY shun):* the ability of the body to convert food to substances suitable for absorption into the blood system.

asteatosis *(AS tee ah TOH sis):* the condition of dry scaly skin, characterized by deficiency of sebum. Asteatosis is usually due to aging or bodily disorders. In local conditions, it may be caused by alkalies, such as those found in soap.

atavistic syndrome *(at ah VIS tik SYN drhom):* syndrome that exhibits hypertrichosis in young girls before puberty.

atom *(AT om):* the smallest component of an element that can exist and still retain the chemical properties of the element.

atopic dermatitis *(AY top ik DER mah TEYE tis):* also known as eczema, a possible hereditary skin disease.

autoclave *(AW toh klayv):* a vessel or chamber producing steam for the sterilization of instruments.

autonomic nervous system *(aw toh NOM ik NUR vus SIS tem):* the part of the nervous system that controls the involuntary muscles.

axilla *(AK sil a):* hair found in the armpit.

axillary *(AK sil er ee):* pertaining to the axilla or armpit.

B

bacilli *(BA sil lee):* rod-shaped bacteria.

bacteria *(bak TEER i ah):* widely distributed unicellular microorganisms with both plant and animal characteristics; the three varieties are bacillus, coccus, and spirillum; some harmful; some are harmless; commonly known as microbes or germs.

bactericide *(bak TEER i seyed):* an agent that destroys bacteria.

bacteriology *(back teer ee OL oh jee):* the science which deals with bacteria.

barba *(BAHR ba):* the growth of beard hair of either men or women.

basal *(BAY sahl):* located at the base which is the lowest or supporting part of anything; lowest or least.

basal cell carcinoma *(BAY sahl sel kahr si NOH mah):* characterized by light or pearly nodules and visible blood vessels.

basal cell epithelioma *(BAY sahl EP i thee lee OH mah):* a raised white spot on the surface of the skin, a cancer caused by exposure to the sun.

benzene *(BEN zeen):* a clear, colorless highly flammable liquid of characteristic odor.

blackhead *(BLAK hed):* also known as a comedone, caused by the hardening of the sebum in the sebaceous gland duct leading to the surface of the skin.

blanching *(BLANCH ing):* whitening of the epidermis. Results from overtreatment with high frequency.

blend current *(blend KUR ent):* alternating current and direct current simulated through a conductor.

blepharoplasty *(BLEF ah roh plas tee):* chemical name for eyelid correction.

bromidrosis *(BROH mi DROH sis):* refers to foul-smelling perspiration, usually noticeable in the armpits or on the feet. Also known as osmidrosis.

bulbous *(BOL bus):* pertaining to or like a bulb in shape and structure.

bulla *(BUL ah):* a blister containing watery fluid, similar to a vesicle, but larger.

C

calamine *(KAL ah meyen):* pinkish powder of zinc oxide and ferric oxide used to treat skin ailments. It is used in electrolysis as an astringent and an anti-irritant.

capillary *(KAP i ler ee):* any one of the minute blood vessels which connect the arteries and veins; hairlike blood vessels.

capilli *(kah PIL lee):* hair, generally referred to as scalp hair.

carbohydrates *(KAR boh HEYE drayts):* substances containing carbon, hydrogen, and oxygen, the two latter in proportion to form water; sugars, starches, and cellulose belong to the class of carbohydrates.

carbon dioxide *(KAHR bon deye OK seyed):* carbonic acid gas; product of the combustion of carbon with a free supply of air. CO_2.

catabolism *(ka TAB o lis em):* the phase of metabolism which involves the breaking down of complex compounds within the cells, often resulting in energy.

catagen phase *(KAT ah jen fays):* the brief transitional period between growth and inactive stage of a hair follicle.

cataphoresis *(KAT ah fo REE sis):* the forcing of substances into the deeper tissues, using the galvanic current from the positive toward the negative pole; the use of the positive pole to introduce an acid pH product such as an astringent solution into the skin. In the skin it can cause hydrochloric acid and disintegrate steel electrolysis needles, causing a permanent black spot. On the surface it will temporarily firm the skin and reduce redness.

cell *(sel):* a living cell must contain a cell wall or cell membrane, protoplasm and a nucleus, forming the structural unit of every organized body; capable of performing all the fundamental functions of life.

cell division *(sel di VIZH zhun):* the reproduction of cells by the process of each cell dividing in half and forming two cells, also known as mitosis.

cell membrane *(sel MEM brayn):* a delicate protoplastic material that encloses a living plant or animal cell; cell wall.

central nervous system *(SEN tral NUR vus SIS tem):* that part of the nervous system in vertebrates which consists of the brain and spinal cord.

cerebro-spinal *(se REE broh-SPEYE nahl):* consists of the brain, spinal cord, spinal nerves and the cranial nerves.

centrosome *(SEN troh sohm):* a cellular body which controls the division of the cell.

chancre *(SHANG ker):* a sore: the primary lesion of syphylis.

characteristic *(kar ik te RIS tik):* a distinguishing trait.

chemical activities *(KEM i kal ak TIV i tees):* activities of the elements.

chemistry *(KEM is tree):* the science which deals with the composition of substances; the elements and their mutual reactions and the phenomena resulting from the formation and decomposition of compounds; the science that deals with the structure and compositional properties of substances and their transformations.

chemotherapy *(kee mo THER a pee):* treatment of the disease cancer, with chemical substances.

chloasma *(kloh AZ mah):* characterized by increased deposits of pigment in the skin found mainly on the forehead, nose and cheeks. Also called moth patches or liver spots.

chlorine *(KLOR een):* a greenish, yellowish gas with a disagreeable, suffocating odor; used in combined form as a disinfectant and bleaching agent.

chronic *(KRON ik):* means long term or even life-long.

chronic disease *(KRON ik di ZEEZ):* is of long duration, usually mild, but recurring.

cilia *(SIL i a):* the eyelashes.

cimetidine *(si MET i deen):* chemical name; also known as Tagament; substance which inhibits gastric acid secretion in response to all stimuli. Presently being tested as an anti-androgen drug to reduce hair growth. Side effects are possibly carcinogenic, and may effect the placenta and maternal milk.

circulation *(sur kyoo LAY shun):* the passage of blood throughout the body.

circulatory system *(SUR kyoo la tohr ee):* the system which carries blood from the heart to all parts of the body and back to the heart, circulating oxygen and nutrients for, and wastes from, the entire body.

club hair *(klub hair):* a non-living hair that is detached from the lower portion of the hair follicle, after the telogen stage. It will eventually fall out due to friction. An anagen hair can possibly be growing beneath it.

coagulation *(koh ag yoo LAY shun):* the process of clot formation; conversion of a fluid into soft jelly-like solid.

cocci *(KOK seye):* spherical cell bacteria appearing singly or in a group.

cold sore *(kold sohr):* herpes simplex; an inflammation of the skin characterized by swollen shiny white or yellowish vessicles, singular or in groups. These infections are contagious. Avoid electrolysis treatment.

collagen *(KOL a jen):* a protein forming the chief constituent of the connective tissues and bones; used in some cosmetics, such as face creams.

connective tissue *(ko NEK tiv TISH oo):* fibrous tissue that unites and supports the various parts of the body such as bone, cartilage or tendons.

colloid *(KOL oid):* a substance consisting of particles having a certain degree of fineness and possessing a sticky consistency; gluey substance.

colloidal *(ko LOY dahl):* being of a gluey substance.

comedones *(kom eh DOH neez):* worm-like masses in obstructed sebaceous ducts.

compound *(KOM pownd):* a substance formed by a chemical union of two or more elements, and different from any of them.

congenital disease *(kahn JEN i tahl di ZEEZ):* is present in an infant at birth.

contact dermatitis *(KON takt dur ma TEYE tis):* inflammation of skin caused by foreign material.

contagious disease *(kahn TAY jus di ZEEZ):* is communicable by contact.

converter *(kon VUR ter):* an apparatus used to convert direct current to alternating current or alternating current to direct current.

cortex *(KOR teks):* the second or middle layer of the hair shaft; the external portion of the adrenal glands.

corticosteroids *(KOR ti ko STE roids):* adrenal cortex hormonal steroid used for its anti-inflammatory properties. Undersecretion of these hormones may cause the pituitary gland to stimulate an overproduction of adrenal androgens, which may cause excess hair growth.

corticotropin-ACTH *(KOR to ko TROH pin):* hormone secreted by anterior pituitary gland. Acts primarily on adrenal cortex by stimulating its growth and secretion of corticosteroids. Releases during times of stress, which can excess hair growth.

cortisone *(KOR ti sohn):* a powerful hormone extracted from the cortex of the adrenal gland and also made synthetically; used in the treatment of disease and some diseases of the skin. When taken as an oral medication, it has been known to cause severe excess hair growth.

crust *(krust):* an accumulation of sebum and pus. The scab on a sore is an example.

crystallized *(KRIS tahl eyezd):* formed into crystals; definite in form.

Cushing syndrome *(COOSH ing SIN drome):* disease characterized by obesity and muscular weakness associated with adrenal or pituitary dysfunction. Causes severe hirsuitism.

cuticle *(KYOO ti kel):* the very thin outer layer of the skin or hair; the epidermis; the crescent of toughened skin around the base of fingernails and toenails; any fine covering.

cyproterone acetate *(seye PROH ter ohn AH se tayt):* a synthetic antiandrogenic steroid; used in treatment of male sexual disorders. Experimentally used to stop hair growth. It's effectiveness and side effects are not fully known.

cysts *(sists):* in general, an abnormally enclosed duct causing a sac or pouch containing a fluid, semifluid or solid; examples are: sebaceous cyst, ovarian cyst, and pilonidal cyst, which usually contains many ingrown hairs.

cystoplasm *(SEYE to plaz em):* all the protoplasm of a cell except that in the nucleus; the watery fluid which nourishes the cell.

D

decomposition *(dee kom po ZISH un):* to separate or disintegrate into constituent parts or elements.

decrepitation *(dee KREP i TAY shun):* the explosion or cracking of certain substances (salts, crystals, etc.) upon heating.

demineralized *(de MIN er al eyezd):* the loss of mineral salts from the body, as from the bones.

demographia *(dem ah GRAF ee ah):* temporary condition. Patient experiences swelling due to scratching or friction of the skin.

depilatories *(di PIL a tohr ees):* substances, usually caustic alkali, that are used to dissolve the hair at the surface of the skin.

dermal papilla *(DUR mal pa PIL a):* an elevation of the projecting corium under the surface of a hair bulb. It contains capillaries through which a hair receives its nourishment. It is not part of the hair follicle.

dermatitis *(dur mah TEYE tis):* is a term used to denote an inflammatory condition of the skin, caused by an allergy.

dermatologist *(dur mah TOL ah jist):* is a skin specialist.

dermatology *(dur mah TOL ah jee):* is the study of skin, its nature, structure and functions, diseases and treatments.

dermis *(DUR mis):* the layer below the epidermis; the corium or true skin. Sometimes known as true skin.

desiccation *(DES i KAY shun):* the process of drying. In electrolysis, bringing the temperature above 212°F.

dexamethosone *(DEK sah METH o sohn):* chemical name; used primarily as an anti-inflammatory in various conditions including the collagen diseases. Administered orally or topically. It is a steroid and may cause excess hair growth.

diabetic *(deye a BET ik):* one who has diabetes, a disease associated with deficient insulin secretion.

diagnosis *(deye ag NOH sis):* is the recognition of a disease from its symptoms.

diaphragm *(DEYE ah fram):* a muscular wall which separates the thorax from the abdominal region and helps to control breathing.

diffusion *(di FYOO zhun):* a spreading out; dialysis.

digestion *(deye JES chun):* the process of converting food into a form which can be readily absorbed; the breaking down of substances into simple forms, as food into simpler chemical compounds.

digestive system *(deye JEST tiv SIS tem):* the internal organs that change food into nutrients and wastes; the alimentary canal with its associated glands.

dimpling *(DIM pling):* the needle is inserted too shallow into the hair follicle. Results from overtreatment on surface and leaves a pit or indentation in the epidermis.

diphtheria *(dif THEER ee a):* an infectious disease in which the air passages and especially the throat, become coated with a false membrane, caused by a specific bacillus.

diplococci *(DIP lo KOK seye):* bacteria that occur in groups of two.

direct current *(DI rekt KUR ent):* "DC"; the electrical current used in the galvanic process of electrolysis.

disease *(di ZEEZ):* any departure from a normal state of health.

disinfect *(dis in FEKT):* to free from infection.

disinfectant *(dis in FEK tant):* the act of freeing one from infection.

distorted hair follicles *(DIS tor ted hair FOL i kels):* follicles that do not grow straight, but curl or bend. Fortunately all hair follicles grow straight in early anagen, and are close to the surface of the skin to allow effective treatment.

dyskeratosis *(DIS ker ah TOH sis):* refers to the imperfect keratinization of individual epidermal cells.

E

eccrine gland *(EK rin gland):* a small sweat gland that is located throughout the surface of the skin of the human body; the glands that produce secretions that are important for heat regulation and hydrating the skin. These glands are found in abundance in the armpit and are not affected by electrolysis treatment.

eczema *(EK ze mah):* inflammatory condition of the skin, either acute or chronic in nature, presenting many forms of dry or moist lesions, frequently accompanied by itching, burning, and various other unpleasant sensations. Requires medical attention.

edema *(eh DEE mah):* is the medical term for swelling.

efferent fibers *(EF er ent FEYE bers):* nerve fibers conveying outward, away from the central nervous system.

elasticity *(EE las TIS i tee):* property of the hair that enables it to retain curl formation and spring back into curled shaped after being extended; important in the ability of hair to retain curl. The skin also has this property which allows the insertion of the needle.

elastin *(i LAS tin):* a protein base similar to collagen, which forms elastic tissue.

electric tweezer *(i LEK trik TWEE zer):* a device which has been claimed to transmit radio frequency (r.f.) energy through the hair shaft into the follicle. The Food and Drug Administration and the Federal Trade Commission question the effectiveness of the device.

electrocoagulation *(i LEEK troh koh AG yoo LAY shun):* using a needle, a high frequency current (short wave) which raises the temperature of the protein within a hair follicle to approximately 107°F to 109°F causing coagulation. This destroys the living tissue of the dermal papilla and lower portion of the follicle, permanently destroying any further hair growth. Also termed (thermolysis).

electrode *(i LEK trohd):* a pole of an electric cell; and applicator for directing the use of electricity on a patient.

electrodesiccation *(i LEK troh DES i KAY shun):* the dehydration of tissue by the use of a high frequency electric current, usually higher than 212°F.

electrolysis *(i lek TROL i sis):* decomposition of a chemical compound or body tissues, particularly hair root protein, by means of electricity and salt water.

element *(EL e ment):* the simplest form of basic matter; a substance that cannot be broken down into a simpler substance without loss of identity.

embedded hair *(em BED ed hair):* See ingrown hair.

emollient *(i MOL yent):* an agent that softens or smooths the surface of the skin.

emulsifier *(i MUL si feye er):* a substance, which helps to keep oils and liquids in suspension to prevent separation of ingredients.

emulsion *(i MUL shun):* substantially permanent mixture of two or more liquids that are normally insoluble and are held in suspension by emulsifiers.

endocrine system *(EN do krin SIS tem):* the ductless glands of the body whose secretions are released directly into the blood stream.

enzyme *(EN zeyem):* a protein compound, capable of accelerating or producing catalytic action to promote a chemical change.

epidemic *(ep i DEM ik):* is the manifestation of a disease that attacks a large number of people, within one locality, simultaneously.

epidermis *(ep i DUR mis):* the outer epithelial portion of the skin.

epilation *(EH pil ay shun):* to remove hair by the root; the hair that is removed after treatment; epilated hair.

epilators *(EH pil ay tors):* electrical medical devices used to epilate hairs permanently.

erythema *(er i THEE mah):* the medical term for redness of the skin.

estrogen *(ES tro jen):* any of various substances that influence estrus or produce changes in the sexual characteristics of females.

ethyl alcohol *(ETH il AL ko hawl):* the basis of some alcoholic beverages; used in cosmetic products, such as astringents, antiseptics and fragrances.

etiology *(ee ti OL ah jee):* is the study of the causes of disease.

excoriation *(eks KOHR ee ay shun):* is a skin sore or abrasion produced by scratching or scraping the raw surface due to the loss of the superficial skin after an injury, for example.

excretion *(ik SKREE shun):* that which is thrown off or eliminated from the body; a substance that is produced by some cells, but in itself is of no further use to the body; the act or process of excreting.

excretory *(EK skre tohr ee):* pertaining to or serving for excretion.

exfoliation *(eks FOH lee AY shun):* peeling and shedding of the horny layer of the skin; a process that normally follows inflammation or occurs in some diseases.

F

factor *(FAK tor):* a circumstance that contributes to a result.

fascia *(FASH ee a):* a fibrous membrane or subcutaneous covering which separates various tissues. It also unites the skin with underlying tissue.

fats *(fahts):* adipose tissues; greasy, soft solid material found in an animal's tissues; plump; obese.

fermentation *(fur men TAY shun):* a chemical decomposition of organic compounds into more simple compounds, brought about by the action of an enzyme.

fertilization *(fur ti li ZAY shun):* the union of the male and female reproductive cells.

fibroblasts *(FEYE broh blasts):* connective tissue cells. Form the fibrous tissues in the body.

filter *(FIL ter):* anything porous through which liquid is passed to cleanse and strain it.

filtration *(fil TRAY shun):* the operation of straining through a filter.

fissure *(FISH yoor):* a crack in the skin penetrating into the dermis, as in the case of the chapped hands or lips.

flagella *(flah JEL la):* a slender whip-like processes which permit locomotion in certain bacteria.

flexible *(FLEK si bel):* capable of being bent; pliable; not stiff.

fluid *(FLOO id):* a non-solid substance; liquid or gas.

follicle *(FOL i kel):* hair follicle; a small secretory cavity or sac; the depression in the skin containing the hair root.

folliculitis *(fah LIK yoo LEYE tis):* when hair follicles become slightly affected and pustules appear, the infection goes deeper and is called folliculitis.

foreign matter *(FOR in MAT ter):* undesirable substance or particle from outside the body, found on or in the skin, hair, nails or body, occurring where they are not normally found. Any foreign matter that enters the hair follicle after electrolysis treatment may cause superficial infection.

formaldehyde *(for MAL de heyed):* a pungent gas possessing powerful disinfectant and preservative.

freckling *(FREK ling):* see hyperpigmentation.

fumigant *(FYOO mi gant):* a gaseous substance capable of destroying pathogenic bacteria.

fundus *(FUN dus):* general term for the bottom or the base.

fungus *(FUN gus):* a vegetable parasite; a spongy growth of diseased tissue on or in the body.

furuncle *(FU rung kel):* also called a boil, is caused by bacteria that enters the skin through the hair follicles. It is a subcutaneous abscess that fills with pus.

fuse *(fyoos):* a safety device placed on an electrical circuit to control the flow of current. If the flow exceeds specifications, the device will blow or break, making a gap in the circuit, causing the flow to stop.

G

galvanic current *(gal VAN ik KUR ent):* see direct current.

galvanic machine, direct current machine *(gal VAN ik ma SHEEN):* an apparatus with attachments designed to produce galvanic current for the permanent removal of unwanted hair, usually with multiple needle holders.

gas *(gahs):* a substance that does not become liquid or solid at ordinary temperatures, that diffuses readily, and that tends to distribute itself evenly throughout an enclosure.

gaseous *(GAS ee us):* of or like a gas.

gastrointestinal *(GAS troh in TES ti nal):* pertaining to both the stomach and intestines.

genetics *(je NET iks):* the science that deals with the heredity and variation of organisms.

germicide *(JUR mi seyed):* any chemical that will destroy germs.

germinative *(jur MI nah tiv):* having the power to grow and develop.

germinative layer *(jur MI nah tiv LAY er):* stratum.

germinativum *(jur MI nah tiv um):* a layer of cells which lies beneath the stratum malpighi and its responsible for the reproduction of new cells of the epidermis.

gland *(gland):* a secretory organ of the body.

globule *(GLOB yools):* small spherical droplets of fluid or semifluid material.

glucocorticoids *(GLOO ko KOR ti koids):* any of the group of corticosteroids predominantly affecting carbohydrate metabolism.

glycerine *(GLIS eh rin):* a colorless, oily substance obtained by hydrolysis of fats and by synthesis; manufactured from the natural substance; glycerol; used as a solvent, emollient, and humectant.

glycogen *(GLEYE ko jen):* animal starch. Large amounts of glycogen are dissolved within the hair follicle. The amount of this solution is directly related to the current levels used in short wave or galvanic electrolysis treatment.

gonadotropin *(GON ah do TROH pin):* any hormone leaving a stimulating effect on the gonads.

gonads *(GOH nads):* primary sex glands; ovaries and testes.

granules *(GRAN yools):* small grains or particles.

growth *(growth):* lengthening of hair, nails, etc.; the process of growing larger; increase in size or maturity; abnormal formation of tissue such as a tumor.

gynecological *(GEYE ne ko LOJ i kahl):* relating to study of female reproductive system and its diseases.

H

hair *(hair):* a slender filament of protein keratin found on most mammals; an appendage or outgrowth of the skin whose root lies in a follicle in the corium and subcutaneous tissue. Only the lower portion of the hair contains living cells.

hair bulb *(hair bulb):* the part of the hair which holds the root; the part which encloses the hair papilla; the lower extremity of the hair.

hair canal *(hair ka NAHL):* the space in the hair follicle occupied by the hair root.

hair root *(hair root):* the part of the hair contained within the follicle.

hair shaft *(hair shaft):* the portion of hair which projects beyond the skin.

Henle's layer *(HEN lees LAY ur):* the outer layer of the inner root sheath.

heredity *(he RED i tee):* the genetic capacity of the organism to develop ancestral characteristics; the transfer of qualities or disease from parents to offspring.

hermaphrodite *(her MAF roh deyet):* an individual who has both male and female sex organs.

hermaphroditism *(her MAF roh deye tizm):* the presence of both male and female sex organs.

herpes simplex *(HUR pees SIM plecks):* fever blister; cold sore.

hirci *(HIR see):* the hairs growing in the axilla.

hirsute *(HER soot):* hairy; having coarse, long hair; shaggy.

hirsutism *(HER soot izm):* a term reserved for females. Refers to growth of hair on face and body which usually is a characteristic of masculinity. It is caused by an overabundance of the hormone androgen.

histology *(hi STOL o jee):* the study of the minute structures of the body.

hormones *(HOR mohns):* secretions produced in and by one of the endocrine glands, such as the pituitary, thyroid, adrenals, etc., and carried by the blood stream or body fluid to another part of the body or body organ to stimulate functional activities. Hormones have a direct or indirect effect on normal and abnormal hair growth.

humectant *(hyoo MEK tant):* a substance which absorbs moisture or promotes retention of moisture; a substance having affinity for water, with the stabilization action on water content of material.

hyalin *(HEYE ah lin):* a translucent substance.

hydrochloric acid *(heye dro KLOHR ik AS id):* a compound of hydrogen and chlorine.

hydrogen *(HEYE dro jen):* the lightest element. An odorless tasteless gas found in water and all organic compounds.

hydrogen peroxide *(HEYE dro jen peh ROK seyed):* a powerful oxidizing agent; in liquid form it is used as an antiseptic, as a neutralizer, and for the activation of lighteners and hair tints; the most common strength for cosmetology use 6% (20% volume).

hyperendrogenism *(HEYE per AN droh jen izm):* too much androgen, which can cause excess hair growth.

hyperemia *(HEYE per EE mee ah):* the presence of an excessive quantity of blood in a part of the body. This could also cause dormant hair follicles to grow hair.

hyperestrogenism *(HEYE per ES troh jen izm):* too much estrogen.

hyperidrosis *(HEYE per i DROH sis):* excessive perspiration caused by intense heat or general body weakness. Most commonly affected parts are armpits, joints, and feet. Requires medical attention.

hyperkeratosis *(heye per KER ah TOH sis):* refers to an abnormal increase in the horny layer of the skin. A callus is an example of this condition.

hyperpigmentation *(HEYE per PIG men TAY shun):* a condition characterized by the production of more melanin in some areas than in others. This condition may result after electrolysis treatment, especially if the area is exposed to the sun. A freckling appearance may occur which could take a few months to a few years to disappear.

hyperthyroidism *(HEYE per THEYE roid izm):* overactive thyroid gland, may cause excess hair growth.

hypertrichosis *(HEYE per treye KOH sis):* excess hair is confined to areas of the arms, legs, feet and sometimes the neck and back; not characterized as masculine.

hypertrophy *(heye PER troh fee):* an excessive growth.

hypoandrogenism *(HEYE poh an DROH jen izm):* too little androgen.

hypoestrogenism *(HEYE poh es TROH jen izm):* too little estrogen.

hypopigmentation *(HEYE poh PIG men TAY shun):* lack of pigment, coloring, of hair, skin etc.

hypothalamus *(HEYE poh THAL ah mus):* the part of the brain that regulates many metabolic processes.

hypothyroidism *(HEYE poh THEYE roid izm):* underactive thyroid gland, may cause excess hair growth.

I

iatrogenic *(eye ah tro JEN ik):* superfluous hair growth caused by drugs.

idiopathic *(id i o PATH ik):* arising from an unknown cause or origin.

immiscible *(i MIS i bel):* unable to be mixed.

immunity *(i MYOO ni tee):* freedom from or resistance to disease.

impetigo *(im pe TEE goh):* an eruption of pustules, caused by staphylococci, which rupture or become crusted, occuring chiefly on the face around the mouth and nostrils. Avoid electrolysis treatment.

infection *(in FEK shun):* the invasion of body tissues by disease germs.

infectious disease *(in FEK shus di ZEEZ)* is due to pathogenic germs taken into the body as a result of contact with an contaminated object or lesion.

infinite *(IN fih nit):* having no limit; endless.

inflammation *(in fla MAY shun):* a condition of some part of the body as a reaction to injury, irritation or infection characterized by redness, heat, pain and swelling.

inflammatory *(in FLAM a tohr ee):* tending to inflame.

ingrown hair *(in GROHN hair):* also known as embedded hair is a hair growing beneath a horny layer of skin. These hairs must be gently lifted out before treatment.

inorganic *(in or GAN ik):* being or composed of matter other than plant or animal; non-carbon.

insoluble *(in SOL yoo bel):* incapable of being dissolved or very difficult to dissolve.

insulator *(in SUH lay tur):* a material that will prevent the flow of electricity.

insulated probe *(in SUH layt ed prohb):* a needle that is surrounded by an insulated material with the exception of its tip.

intensity *(in TEN si tee):* the amount of force per unit area, as of heat, light or current; the quality of being intense.

intensity control *(in TEN si tee kon TROL):* regulates current flow (rheostat).

intercellular *(in ter SEL yoo lar):* between or among cells.

intermediate hair *(in ter MEE di it hair):* the hair that is between the vellus and terminal hair.

irritability *(ir i ta BIL i tee):* the quality or state of being readily excited or stimulated to annoyance.

isolate *(EYE so layt):* to set apart from others.

K

keloids *(KEE loids):* thick scars resulting from excessive growth of fibrous tissue, making the scar larger than the original wound or treated area; a concern in electrology treatment, especially with negroid peoples.

keloid acne *(KEE loid AK nee):* a follicular infection with pustules which cause keloidal scarring; frequently affects black skin.

keratin *(KER a tin):* a fiber protein characteristic of horny tissues: hair, nails, feathers, etc.; it is insoluble in protein solvents and has a high sulfur content; the principal constituent of hair and nails.

keratoma *(KER ah TOH mah):* (or callus) is a thickened patch of epidermis, caused by friction, usually on the hands and feet.

keratosis *(ker ah TOH sis):* any disease of the epidermis that is marked by the presence of circumscribed overgrowths of the horny layer.

L

lanugo *(lah NOO goh):* the fine hair, covering the body, which is present at birth.

laser *(LAY zer):* an instrument that emits radiation as a beam of great power; used in surgical procedures and research, and presently being tested for electrology treatment.

lentigines *(len TIJ i neez):* (lentigo—singular), or freckles, are small yellowish-to-brownish colored spots on parts of the body exposed to sunlight and air.

lesion *(LEE zhun):* a primary or secondary infection, injury or disease to the skin.

leucoderma *(LOO koh DER mah):* refers to abnormal patches of light skin due to congenital pigmentation.

lice *(leyes):* plural of louse; animal parasites that infest the hairs of the head.

licensure *(LEYE sen shur):* the granting of licenses to practice a profession.

litmus *(LIT muhs):* strips of paper containing color matter used in testing acidity or alkalinity of a product; red turns blue to indicate alkalinity and blue turns red to indicate acidity.

lordosis *(lor DOH sis):* a forward curvature of the lumbar spine, swayback.

louse *(lows):* singular of lice; animal parasite that infests the hairs of the head. Electrolysis treatment must be avoided.

lye *(leye):* a chemical known as (NaOH) sodium hydroxide; it is the chemical in solution that is created by the galvanic method of electrolysis, that causes the permanent destruction of the tissue causing hair growth.

lymph *(limf):* a clear, yellowish fluid which circulates in the lymph spaces (lymphatics) of the body.

lymph crusts *(limf crusts):* appear as light colored scabs after electrolysis treatment more so on the body than the face. They fall off within a few days.

lymph-vascular *(limf-VAS kyoo lar):* drainage system for the body tissues.

lymphatic *(lim FAT ik):* pertaining to, containing, or conveying lymph.

lymphocyte *(LIM foh ceyet):* a colorless weakly motil cell produced in lymphoid tissue that is the typical cellular element of lymph and constitues 20 to 30 percent of the leucocytes of normal human blood.

M

macule *(MAK yool):* small discolored spot or patch on a surface of the skin, not raised, and not sunken; a freckle.

magnesium sulfate *(mag NEE zee um SUL fayt):* an ingredient used in medicinal preparations and in some shampoos formulated for oily hair.

malignant melanoma *(mah LIG nant mel ah NOH mah):* characterized by (dark brown, black, or discolored) patches on the skin.

malphigian *(mal PIG i an):* middle layer of the wall of the primitive neural tube containing primitive nerve cells and later forming the gray substance of the central nervous system.

matrix *(MAY triks):* the formative portion of a nail or a tooth; the intercellular substance of a tissue.

matter *(MAT er):* substance that occupies space and has weight.

medicament *(me DIK a meant):* a medicinal substance or agent.

medicamentosus *(MED i kah men TOH sus):* a skin eruption caused by a drug.

medicinal *(meh DI si nahl):* having healing properties.

medulla *(mi DUL al):* the pitch of the hair; the marrow in the various bone cavities; soft inner portion of an organ.

megahertz *(MEG a hurts):* a unit of frequency, equaling one million cycles per second.

meiosis *(meye OH sis):* special method of cell division, occurring in maturation of the sex cells, by means of which each daughter nucleus receives half the number of chromosomes characteristic of the somatic cells of the species.

melanin *(MEL ah nin):* the dark pigment in the epidermis and hair and in the choroid or coat of the eye.

melanocyte *(MEL ah non seyet):* a melanin-forming cell.

melanoma *(MEL ah noh mah):* generally, a bluish black shiny lesion; it is irregular in shape and contains no hair growth. They can become malignant, especially if they increase in size, bleed, or look irritated.

membrane *(MEM brayn):* a thin sheet or layer of pliable tissue surrounding a part separating adjacent cavities, lining a cavity, or connecting adjacent structures.

menarche *(me NAHR kee):* the beginning of the menstrual function; the first menstrual function.

metabolism *(me TAB o liz em):* the constructive and destructive life process of the cell.

metamorphosis *(met ah MOR foh sis):* change of physical form, structure or substance.

metaphase *(MET ah fayz):* in biology (cell division), the middle state in mitosis when chromosomes become aligned in the middle of the spindle.

microscopic *(meye kro SKOP ik):* extremely small; visible only with the aid of a microscope; not visible to the naked eye.

miliaria rubra *(mil ee AH rah ROO brah):* prickly heat. It is an acute inflammation of the sweat glands characterized by small, red vessicles and accompanied by burning and itching of the skin. It is caused by exposure to excessive heat and obesity.

milia *(MIL ee ah):* a whitehead; small whitish pearlike mass in the epidermis due to the retention of sebum.

milliampere *(MIL i AM peer):* one thousandth of an ampere.

milliameter *(mil ee AM e ter):* an instrument which registers electric current in milliamperes; used to measure the amount of current required for a given treatment.

milliamperemeter *(MIL i am PEER mee tur):* a milliameter; an instrument that measures milliamperes, or measures current in thousandths of an ampere.

miscible *(MIS ih bel):* able to be mixed.

mitosis *(meye TOH sis):* indirect nuclear division, the usual process of cell reproduction of human tissue.

mixtures *(MIKS churs):* preparation made by incorporating an insoluble ingredient in a liquid vehicle; sometimes used to identify an aqueous solution containing two or more solutes; a combination of two or more substances which are not chemically united.

modality *(moh DAHL i tee):* is the term used to designate one of the three acceptable methods of permanent hair removal: electrolysis, thermolysis, or the combination of both.

moisturizer *(MOYS chu reyez er):* a product formulated to add moisture to dry skin or hair.

mole *(mohl):* a macule that is tan to dark brown in color that may or may not contain hair. Electrologist must check with insurance company before treatment.

molecule *(MOL eh kyool):* the smallest possible unit of any substance that still retains its characteristics.

muscular *(MUS kyoo lar):* relating to a muscle or the muscles.

myology *(meye OL o jee):* the science of the nature, functions, structure and diseases of muscles.

N

nerve *(nurv):* a whitish cord, made up of bundles of nerve fibers through which impulses are transmitted.

nervous system *(NUR vus SIS tem):* the body system composed fo the brain, spinal cord, nerves, ganglia and other parts of the receptors.

neuro-transmitters *(noor oh-trans MIT urs):* a substance that transmits nerve impulses across a synapse.

neurology *(noo ROL o jee):* the science of the structure, function and pathology of the nervous system.

neuron *(NOOR on):* the basic unit of the nervous system, consisting of a nucleus, its processes and extensions; a nerve cell.

neutral *(NOO tral):* exhibiting no positive properties; neither acid nor alkaline.

neutrality *(noo TRAL i tee):* the state of being neutral.

neutralize *(NOO tral eyez):* to render ineffective; counterbalance of an action or influence.

nevus *(NEE vus):* a birthmark; malformations of the skin due to pigmentation or dilated capillaries, sometimes hairy.

nitrates *(NEYE trayts):* an oxidizing agent.

nitrogen *(NEYE troh jen):* a colorless, gaseous element, tasteless and odorless, found in air and living tissue.

nonpathogenic *(NON path o JEN ik):* not harmful; not disease producing.

nucleus *(NOO klee us):* the active center of cells.

nutriment *(NOO tri ment):* that which nourishes; food.

nutrition *(noo TRISH on):* the processes involved in taking in nutriments and assimilation and utilizing them.

O

obese *(oh BEES):* extremely overweight; stout; corpulent; fat.

objective *(ob JEK tiv):* refers to symptoms that can be seen, such as pimples, pustules or inflammation.

occupational disease *(ok yoo PAY shuh nahl di ZEEZ)* : such as dermatitis, is due to certain kinds of employment and is caused by coming in contact with cosmetic chemicals, detergents, etc.

Ohm's Law *(ohms law):* is a measurement of electrical resistance, or voltage equals current times resistance.

ointment *(OYNT ment):* a medicated mixture applied externally; a preparation for the skin or scalp.

organ *(OR gan):* in plants and animals, a structure composed of specialized tissues and performing specific functions.

organic chemistry *(or GAN ik KEM is tree):* chemistry of carbon compounds.

organism *(OR gah niz em):* any animal or plant with organs that function to maintain life.

organization *(OR hag ni ZAY shun):* the act or process of organizing or being organized.

oscillation *(OS i LAY shun):* movement like a pendulum, a swinging or vibrating.

oscillator *(OS i LAY tohr):* an apparatus that produces vibrating movements used in massage.

osmidrosis *(oz mi DROH sis):* refers to foul-smelling perspiration, usually noticeable in the armpits or on the feet. Also known as bromidrosis.

osmosis *(oz MOH sis):* the diffusion of a fluid or solution through a semipermeable membrane: especially the passage of a solvent through a membrane from a dilute solution into a more concentrated one.

osteology *(os tee OL a jee):* the science of the anatomy structure, and function of bones.

outer root sheath *(ow tur root sheeth):* is the covering of the follicle wall. It contains most of the moisture which is directly related to the current intensity the electrologist must use.

ovarian *(oh VAIR ee an):* or, relating to or, or involving an ovary.

ovaries *(OH vah reez):* plural of ovary; see ovary.

ovary *(OH vah ree):* the essential female reproductive organ that produces eggs and sex hormones.

ovum *(OH vum):* a female gamete.

oxide *(OK seyed):* a compound of oxygen with another element.

oxygen *(OK si jen):* a gaseous element; essential to animal and plant life.

P

pain receptors *(payn ree SEP torz):* sensory nerve fibers that respond to pain-causing stimuli.

pancreas *(PAN kree as):* a gland located in the abdomen that secretes an enzyme that digests proteins, fats, carbohydrates, and the hormone insulin.

papilla *(pah PIL ah):* a small, cone-shaped elevation at the bottom of the hair follicle. (see dermal papilla).

papillae *(pa PIL ee):* singular of papilla.

papillary *(PAP i ler ee):* relating to, resembling, or provided with papillae.

papillary layer *(PAP i ler ee LAY er):* the outer layer of the dermis.

papule *(PAP yool):* small, elevated pimple in the skin. It contains no fluid, but may develop pus.

parakeratosis *(PAHR ah ker ah TOH sis):* refers to nuclei in the cells of the horny layer of the skin.

parasite *(PAR a seyet):* a vegetable or animal organism which lives in or on another organism and draws its nourishment from that organism.

parasitic disease *(par ah SIT ik di ZEEZ):* is produced by disease-producing bacteria, such as staphylococcus and streptococcus, which are pus-forming bacteria.

parathyroid gland *(par ah THEYE roid gland):* small endocrine gland located in or near the thyroid gland. Produces a hormone concerned with calcium metabolism.

pathogenic *(path o JEN ik):* causing disease; disease producing.

pathology *(pah THOL o jee):* is the study of disease.

pediculosis *(pe DIK yoo LOH sis):* a skin disease caused by infestation of lice.

pellegra *(peh LEG grah):* a result of severe vitamin B deficiency which shows a characteristic skin rash that can cause scarring.

pericardium *(per i CAHR dee um):* the membraneous sac around the heart.

peripheral nervous system *(pe RIF er rahl NUR vus SIS tem):* system of nerves and ganglia that connect the peripheral parts of the body to the central nervous system; it has both sensory nerves and motor nerves.

permeable *(PUR mee ah bel):* permitting the passage of liquids.

pharmaceutical *(fahr mah SOO ti kahl):* for or engaged in pharmacy or medicine.

pharmacy *(FAHR mah see):* the preparation and dispensing of medicinal drugs.

pharynx *(FAH rinks):* the upper portion of the digestive tube behind the nose and mouth.

pheromones *(FER o mohns):* a chemical substance that is produced by an animal to serve as a stimulus to other animals of the same species for a behavioral response.

phoresis *(foh REE sis):* a combining form meaning transmission; the process of introducing solutions into tissues through the skin by use of galvanic current.

photoepilator *(foh toh EP i LAY tur):* a device using a portion of the light spectrum. It's effectiveness in hair removal is questionable.

physiological *(FIZ i o LOJ i kahl):* of or relating to the functions of an organism and its parts during life.

physiology *(fiz i OL o jee):* the science of the functions of living things and their parts.

pigment *(PIG ment):* any organic coloring matter; as that of the red blood cells, the hair, skin, iris, etc.

pigmentation *(pig men TAY shun):* the deposition of pigment in the skin or tissues.

pili-multigemini *(pil ee MUHL tee JEM i neye):* several hairs growing from a single follicle opening.

pilonidal *(pil oh NEYE dahl):* hair-containing cavity which often opens at a post anal dimple, containing an accumulation of hairs in a cyst.

pilosebaceous *(PEE lo se BAY shus):* pertaining to the hair follicles and the sebaceous glands together.

pimple *(PIMP pel):* any small pointed elevation of the skin; a papule or small pustule.

pituitary gland *(pi TOO i ter ee gland):* a ductless gland located at the base of the brain.

placenta *(pla SEN tah):* the nourishing substance surrounding an embryo or fetus; after birth; used in some facial preparations.

pliability *(pleye ah BIL i tee):* flexibility.

polarities *(poh LAR i teez):* two opposite poles, as that possessed by a magnet or electric current; plus or minus; positive or negative.

polycystic *(POL ee SIS tik):* containing or made up of many cysts.

pore *(pohr):* a small opening of the sweat glands of the skin.

porosity *(po ROS i tee):* ability of the hair to absorb moisture or liquids.

prednisone *(PRED ni sohn):* synthetic glucocorticoid derived from cortisone.

prognosis *(prog NOH sis):* is the foretelling of the probable course of a disease.

prophase *(PROH fayz):* the first state in mitosis.

protein *(PROH teen):* a complex organic substance present in all living tissue, such as skin, hair and nails; necessary to sustain life; also used in some skin and hair conditioners.

protoplasm *(PROH toh plaz em):* the material basis of life; a substance found in all living cells.

pruritus *(pru REYE tis):* is the medical term for a skin inflammation that causes itching.

psoriasis *(so REYE ah sis):* a skin disease characterized by red patches; covered with adherent white-silver scales.

puberty *(PYOO ber tee):* period of becoming first capable of reproducing sexually; development of secondary sex characteristics.

pubes *(pyoobs):* pubic hair.

pus *(pus):* a fluid product of inflammation, consisting of a liquid containing leucocytes and debris of dead cells and tissue elements.

pustule *(PUS chool):* en elevation of the skin which has an inflamed base and contains pus.

Q

quaternary ammonium compounds *(KWAH ter nah ree ah MOH nee um CAHM pownds):* a group of compounds of organic salts of ammonia employed very effectively as disinfectants, conditioners and other surface-active agents.

R

radio frequency *(RAY dee oh FREE kwen see):* any of the electromagnetic frequencies between those of the audible range and the infrared range.

rectifier *(REK ti feye er):* an apparatus to change an alternating current of electricity into a direct current.

regenerate *(re JEN e rayt):* formed or created again. If the dermal papilla during electroloysis treatment is not totally destroyed, it may regenerate into another papilla, causing new hair growth in the same hair follicle.

regrowth *(REE growth):* for whatever reason, the growth of a new hair, from a follicle that has had electrology treatment.

regulate *(REG yoo layt):* to bring order, method, or uniformity.

repair *(ri PAIR):* to fix; to restore to a healthy state.

reproduction *(ree pro DUK shun):* the process by which plants and animals produce offspring.

reproductive *(ree pro DUK tiv):* pertaining to reproduction or the process by which plants and animals produce offspring.

respiration *(res pi RAY shun):* the act of breathing; the process of inhaling air into the lungs and expelling it.

respiratory *(RES pi rah tohr ee):* relation to respiration.

reticular *(re TIK yoo lar):* sponge-like structure associated with the medulla of the hair and the lower layer of the dermis.

rheostat *(REE o stat):* a resistance coil; an instrument used to regulate the strength of an electric current or intensity of light.

rhinoplasty *(REYE no plas tee):* commonly known as a nosejob.

rhytidectomy *(rit i DEK toh mee):* clinical name for a face-lift.

rosacea *(roh ZAY shee ah):* is associated with excessive oiliness of the skin, chronic redness, dilation of the blood vessels, and the formation of papules and pustules; skin becomes coarse and the scores enlarge.

S

sacral *(SA kral):* pertaining to or located near the sacrum; the five fused vertebrae in humans.

sanitary *(SAN i tee ree):* pertaining to cleanliness in relation to health, or to the absence of any agent that may be injurious to health.

sanitation *(san i TAY shun):* the maintenance of sanitary conditions to promote hygiene and the prevention of disease.

sanitize *(SAN i teyez):* to make sanitary.

sanitizer *(SAN i teyez er):* a chemical agent or product used to sanitize implements; a tall glass or plastic jar filled with a sanitizing agent in which implements are kept in a sanitary condition.

saprophyte *(SAP roh feyet):* a microorganism which grows normally on dead matter, as distinguished from a parasite.

saturated *(SACH u rayt ed):* to become soaked or completely penetrated.

scab *(skab):* a crust of hardened blood serum and dead cells formed over the surface of a wound.

scabies *(SKAY bees):* a skin disease caused by an animal parasite, accompanied by intense itching.

scale *(skayl):* an accumulation of epidermal flakes. Scales can be dry or greasy, such as abnormal or excessive dandruff.

scar *(skahr):* hardened tissue which forms over injuries that penetrate the dermis.

scoliosis *(SKOH lee OH sis):* abnormal lateral curvature of the spine.

scurvy *(SKUR vee):* a disease that produces skin lesions.

seasonal disease *(SEE zuh nahl di ZEEZ):* is influenced by the weather as prickly heat in summer and forms of eczema which are more prevalent in cold weather.

sebaceous gland *(si BAY shus gland):* oil gland of the skin; any gland in the corium of the skin that secretes sebum.

seborrhea *(seb o REE ah):* is a skin condition caused by over-activity of the sebaceous glands.

seborrheic dermatitis *(SEB o REE ik dur mah TEYE tis):* dandruff.

seborrheic keratosis *(SEB o REE ik ker ah TOH tis):* benign skin lesion.

sebum *(SEE bum):* the fatty or oil secretions of the sebaceous glands.

secretion *(se KREE shun):* the process by which materials are separated from the blood usually by glandular function, and formed into new substances used to carry out special functions.

sensation *(sen SAY shun):* a feeling or impression arising as the result of the stimulation of an afferent nerve.

sepsis *(SEP sis):* the presence of various pus-forming and other pathogenic organisms, or their toxins, in the blood or tissues.

sheath *(sheeth):* a covering enclosing or surrounding some organ.

skin disease *(skin di ZEEZ):* is an infection of the skin characterized by an objective lesion (one which can be seen), which may consist of scales, pimples, or pustules.

skeletal muscles *(SKEL e tal MUS sels):* muscles connected to the skeleton.

skin *(skin):* external covering of the body, and largest organ of the human body.

sodium bicarbonate *(SOH dee um beye KAHR bo nit):* a white crystalline, weakly alkaline salt; baking soda.

sodium borate *(SOH dee um BOHR ayt):* a weak, antibacterial and astringent borax.

sodium chloride *(SOH dee um KLOHR eyed):* a powerful alkaline product used in some chemical hair relaxers; caustic soda; powerful alkali used in the manufacturing of liquid soaps.

soluble *(SOL yoo bel):* capable of being dissolved.

solute *(SOL yoot):* a dissolved substance.

solvent *(SOL vent):* able to dissolve another substance.

sperm *(sperm):* a male gamete; seed.

spherical *(SFEER i kahl):* relating to or having the shape of a sphere.

spireme *(SPI reem):* continuous thread-like figure formed by chromosome material during the prophase of mitosis and meiosis.

spirilla *(spi RIL ah):* spiral bacteria.

spironolactone *(SPEYE roh noh LAK tohn):* is a diuretic drug that blocks the sodium-retaining action of aldostrone.

spongiosis *(spun jee OH sis):* is a condition that produces a sponge-like appearance of the skin due to an increase of fluid in the cell layers.

squamous cell cancer *(SKWA mus sel KAN ser):* scaly; covered with scales; thin and flat, like fish's scales.

stain *(stayn):* an abnormal discoloration remaining after the disappearance of moles, freckles, or liver spots, sometimes after certain diseases.

staphylococci *(STAF i lo KOK seye):* cocci which are grouped in clusters like a bunch of grapes; found in pustules and boils.

steatoma *(stee ah TOH mah):* (or wen); is a subcutaneous tumor of the sebaceous glands. It ranges in size from a pea to an orange and consists of sebum. It usually occurs on the scalp, neck, or back.

Stein-Leventhal syndrome *(Steyen-Lev en tahl SIN drome):* multiple cysts of the ovary, causing abnormal menstruation and hirsutism.

sterile *(STER il):* free from all living organisms.

sterilization *(ster i li ZAY shun):* the process of making sterile; the destruction of germs.

sterilize *(STER i leyez):* to deprive of production power; to make sterile or free from microorganisms.

stimuli *(STIM yoo leye):* things that rouse or incite activity.

stratum corneum *(STRA tum KOR nee um):* horny layer of the skin.

stratum germinativum *(STRA tum jur mu nah TIV um):* the deepest layer of the epidermis resting on the corneum.

stratum granulosum *(STRA tum gran yoo LOH sum):* granular layer of the skin.

stratum lucidum *(STRA tum LOO si dum):* the clear, transparent layer of the epidermis under the stratum corneum.

stratum malphigii *(STRA tum mal PIG EE):* the germinative or innermost layer of the epidermis including the spinosum or prickle layer.

stratum mucosum *(STRA tum myoo KOH sum):* mucous or malphigian layer of the skin.

stratum spinosum *(STRA tum spi NOH sum):* the prickle cell layer of the skin often classified with the stratum germinativum to form the basal layer; prickle-like threads join the cells.

streptococci *(STREP to KOK seye):* pus-forming bacteria that arrange in curved lines resembling a string of beads; found in erysipelas and blood poisoning.

structure *(STRUK chur):* the action of building; something arranged in a definite pattern of organization.

subcutaneous *(sub kyoo TAY nee us):* under the skin.

subcutis *(sub KYOO tis):* subdermis; subcutaneous tissue; under or beneath the corium or dermis; the true skin.

suderiferous glands *(SOO do RIF er us):* sweat glands of the skin.

subjective *(sub JEK tiv):* symptoms that can be felt, such as itching, burning, or pain.

superficial *(soo per FISH al):* pertaining to or being on the suface.

superfluous hair *(soo PUR floo us):* more than is required, excessive; unwanted hair.

suprarenal *(SOO prah REE nahl):* situated above or anterior to the kidneys.

suspension *(su SPEN shun):* a state of matter in which the solid particles are dispersed in or distributed throughout a liquid medium; the particles in the medium are large, but not large enough to settle to the bottom under the influence of gravity.

symptom *(SIMP tom):* sign of disease.

synapse *(SIN aps):* the point at which a nervous impulse passes from one neuron to another.

sympathetic nervous system *(sim pah THET ik NUR vus SIS tem):* the part of the autonomic nervous system concerned with mediating involuntary responses of the body such as heart rate, salivary secretion, blood pressure, digestion, etc.

syphilis *(SIF i lis):* a serious disease that is transmitted through sexual contact.

systemic disease *(si STEM ik di ZEEZ):* is due to under- or overfunctioning of the internal glands. It may be caused by faulty diet.

T

tactile corpuscle *(TAK til KOR puh sel):* small epidermal structures with nerve endings that are sensitive to touch and pressure.

tagament *(TAG ah met):* trademark for preparations of cimetidine.

telogen *(TEL oh jen):* the final resting phase of the hair cycle in a follicle, lasting until the fully grown hair is shed, at which time anagen begins. The terminal hair or club hair at this time requires no nourishment and will eventually shed itself by friction, such as brushing or combing.

telophase *(TEL oh fayz):* the final stage of mitosis in which the chromosomes reorganize to form an interstage nucleus.

terminal hair *(TUR mi nal):* tertiary hair; the long, soft hair found on the scalp also present on legs, arms, and body of both males and females.

tertiary *(TUR shee er ee):* third in rank order or formation.

testes *(TES teez):* male gonads that produce male reproductive cells and the male sex hormone testosterone.

testosterone *(tes TOS te rohn):* male sex hormone.

thermolysis *(thur MOL i sis):* the use of high frequency or short-wave current to remove superfluous hair.

thyroid gland *(THEYE royd gland):* a large ductless gland situated in from and on either side of the trachea: it produces the hormone thyroxine which regulates the growth and metabolism of the body; hyper- (too much) or hypo- (too little) thyroidism may cause excess hair growth.

thyroxin *(theye ROK sin):* a hormone secreted by the thyroid gland; the gland regulating body metabolism.

topical *(TOP i kahl):* pertaining to the surface.

tragi *(TRAY je):* hair growing on the pinna of the external ear.

trait *(trayt):* a distinguishing quality; inherited characteristic.

transformer *(trans FOR mer):* a device used for increasing or decreasing the voltage of the current used; it can only be used on an alternating current.

trichology *(tri KOL o jee):* is the study of hair, its diseases, and care.

tubercule *(TOO ber kel):* a solid lump, larger than a papule. It can project above the surface, lie within, or lie under the skin.

tumors *(TOO mors):* are abnormal growths of swollen tissue that can be located on any part of the body.

typhoid *(TEYE foyd):* acute, infectious fever with intestinal lesions and an eruption of rose-colored spots on the chest and abdomen.

tweezing *(TWEE zing):* the temporary removal of hair by simply pulling.

U

ulcer *(UL ser):* an open lesion on the skin or mucous membrane of the body accompanied by pus or loss of skin depth.

V

vascular *(VAS kyoo lar):* supplied with blood vessels; pertaining to a vessel for the conveyance of a fluid, such as blood or lymph.

vellus *(VEL us):* the fine, downy light-colored hair that appears on the body with the exception of the palms of the hands and soles of the feet; they grow from very shallow hair follicles.

veneral disease *(ve NEER ee al di ZEEZ):* is a contagious disease which is contracted during sexual intercourse with an infected person.

verruca *(ve ROO kah):* technical term for wart; it is a viral infection of the epidermis.

vesicle *(VES i kel):* a blister containing clear fluid. A vesicle can be within or just beneath the epidermis.

vibrissae *(vi BRIS ay):* nostril hair; not to be treated by the electrologist.

virilism *(VIR i lizm):* development of secondary sex characteristics in a male at an early age; the appearance of secondary male characteristics in the female.

vitiligo *(VIT i LEE goh):* milky-white spots of the skin.

volatile *(VOL ah til):* evaporates rapidly.

W

wart *(wort):* verruca; thickened epidermis, tumor-like, caused by virus.

watt *(wat):* measures electrical power; watts equal amperes times volts.

waxing *(WAKS ing):* refers to soft wax used to remove hair temporarily; mass tweezing.

wen *(wen):* a sebaceous cyst; usually on the scalp.

wheal *(hweel):* an itchy, swollen lesion that lasts only a few hours. Hives, or the bite of an insect are good examples.

white corpuscles *(weyet KOR pus sels):* (or leucocytes), these cells are found in the blood stream and are the body's defense system against infection and disease.

Index